PURE
SKIN

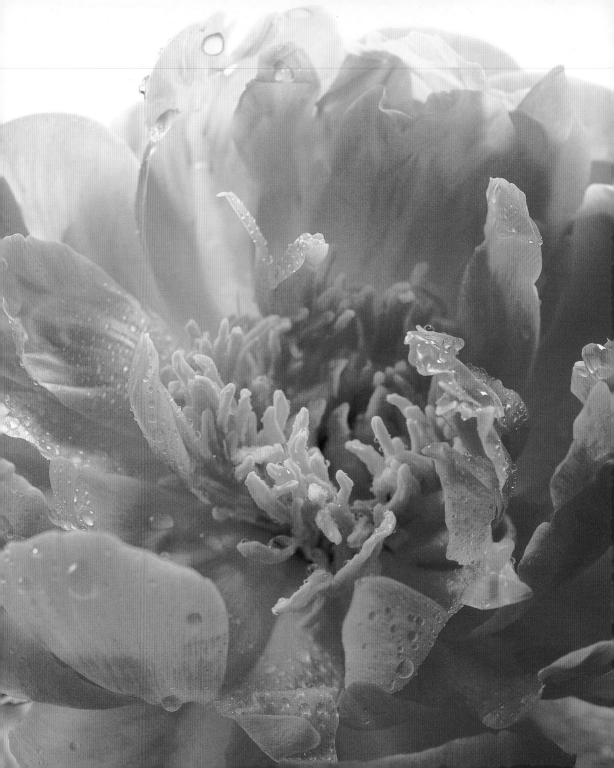

PURE SKIN
ORGANIC BEAUTY BASICS

BARBARA CLOSE

PHOTOGRAPHS BY GENTL & HYERS / EDGE

CHRONICLE BOOKS
SAN FRANCISCO

DEDICATION

To my beloved father

ACKNOWLEDGMENTS

My deepest appreciation to all of the staff of Naturopathica, whose hard work, dedication, and determination to beat the odds are truly the inspiration behind this book. I would also like to thank Lisa Campbell and Mikyla Bruder at Chronicle Books for their guidance.

Text copyright © 2005 by Barbara Close.
Photographs copyright © 2005 by Gentl & Hyers.
All rights reserved. No part of this book may be reproduced
in any form without written permission from the publisher.

Library of Congress Cataloging-in-Publication
Data available.

ISBN 0-8118-4348-3

Manufactured in China

Design by Julia Flagg

Distributed in Canada by Raincoast Books
9050 Shaughnessy Street
Vancouver, British Columbia V6P 6E5

10 9 8 7 6 5 4 3 2 1

Chronicle Books LLC
85 Second Street
San Francisco, California 94105

www.chroniclebooks.com

CONTENTS

INTRODUCTION

To be perfectly honest, I am the last person I would ever expect to end up working in the health and beauty industry. First, I did not begin what I would call a "skin-care regimen" until I was well past college. Second, I am far too passionate about good food and wine to ever conceive of being a purist. And, frankly, I've always been put off by what I perceive as the extremist, or "holier than thou," attitude of some health enthusiasts.

I have a favorite saying that I often repeat to clients: "Everything in moderation—even moderation." If you enjoy steak, have one (preferably organic). You shouldn't have steak every day, but you can certainly eat it every so often. In fact, I think it is the psychology of deprivation and radical self-imposed restraint that causes so many people to fall off the wagon and use unhealthy coping mechanisms like overeating junk food, binge drinking, and other compulsive behaviors.

When I founded my company, Naturopathica Holistic Health, my goal was to educate people about natural health, wellness, and beauty in a new and exciting way. I wanted to define beauty and well-being not as an end in itself but as a means to living a realistic, healthy, and vibrant life that reflects one's beauty from the inside out.

The problem with the concept of beauty today is that it relies on quick fixes like Botox, plastic surgery, and the latest "miracle cream," so the results remain only skin deep. The factors that cause our face and body to age are not being considered. As I see it, feeling beautiful is no longer about "beauty secrets." Instead, beauty is the confidence that makes a woman feel comfortable in her own skin. This type of beauty is not about shoring up on the outside and looking for "hope in a jar." It is about being at home on the inside, a genuine *organic* beauty.

This is the essence of holistic skin care, the basis of this book. Holistic skin care makes you an active participant in promoting your own skin's health by supporting your body's natural healing process. This skin-care method is based on the following core principles of naturopathic medicine:

THE HEALING POWER OF NATURE. This principle is grounded in the belief that the body has an innate ability to heal itself and promote vitality if given the proper support to the immune, circulatory, and lymphatic systems of the body.

DO NO HARM. Holistic skin care never uses raw materials that would be detrimental to the health of the individual.

TREAT THE CAUSE. Skin imbalances are different for each individual. Until the causative factors have been addressed, the condition cannot be effectively treated.

HOLISTIC APPROACH. This approach assumes that skin disturbances have multiple origins, affecting mind, body, and spirit, each of which must be addressed.

Pure Skin is designed to show you how to practice holistic skin care and radiate this inner beauty, providing all the inspiration, resources, and practical advice that you will need. The beauty tips and natural health practices that you are about to learn reflect the more than twenty years of experience

I have had as a natural health practitioner and are designed to educate and assist you in using nutritional medicine, aromatherapy, herbal remedies, massage, water cures, and mind-body techniques to transform how you look and feel from the inside out.

As I wrote this book, my challenge was to present these rituals in the context of how we really live. In today's world, where the concept of multi-tasking is highly prized, how do we find the time, let alone the capability, to sit and meditate with single focus? With most of us balancing both a career and a family, how do we find stamina to create rituals that nourish the body instead of depleting it? My goal was to create a path to healthy beauty that takes into consideration the world that we live in.

The first chapter, **"THE SKIN YOU'RE IN: A USER'S MANUAL,"** focuses on the fundamentals of skin but moves beyond the usual skin typing (normal/dry/oily) to help you better understand your skin. This section views the skin from a holistic approach and explores how problems such as acne, rosacea, and dry skin are reflections of imbalances on a deeper level: emotional, spiritual, or physiological. This chapter will give you an understanding of the various skin personalities, which will help you develop personalized skin-care routines—your beauty basics.

The power of plant materials to improve the health of your skin is explored in chapter 2, **"PURE INGREDIENTS, PURE RESULTS: SKIN-CARE RECIPES."** This section cuts through the hype and marketing of the beauty industry to give you the bottom line on harmful ingredients in skin-care products. You'll learn about the toxicity of many common over-the-counter cosmetic ingredients and how to read a cosmetic label. Next, the active benefits of essential oils, pure vegetal oils, plant enzymes, and botanical extracts are explained, so you can know what to look for when you shop for healthy skin-care products. This chapter goes one step farther by showing you techniques for blending aromatherapy ingredients and recipes for even the most difficult skin-care problems, so you can create your own natural skin-care products at home.

We are all too familiar with the adage "You are what you eat." Nevertheless, succumbing to convenience foods that are empty of nutrients and make us look and feel bad seems inevitable. Chapter 3, **"DETOX AND RETOX: EATING FOR BEAUTIFUL SKIN,"** will help you to recognize the key signs of toxic overload and develop a detox plan—the first step toward healing your skin and body. Then, by eating delicious, nutritionally rich foods, you will nourish your skin internally, thereby slowing down the body's natural aging process. More important, these foods will also help sustain you when the inevitable "retox" phase begins again—that is, when you fall back into unhealthy habits.

The final chapter, **"BEAUTY IN BALANCE: RESTORATIVE THERAPIES,"** shows how to use many of the staples of natural healing to create a whole new way of living—a lifestyle based on returning to balance. This chapter demonstrates how herbs, massage, and energetic medicines—homeopathy and flower essences—can maximize your skin fitness and overall well-being.

The essence of beauty lies within: when we feel our best, we look our best. *Pure Skin* is your beauty and well-being workbook, to make looking after yourself easier and more pleasurable throughout every stage in your life. Ultimately, beauty is an attitude, an approach to living. *Pure Skin* will make it simple to embrace your essential beauty secret: living well is the best revenge.

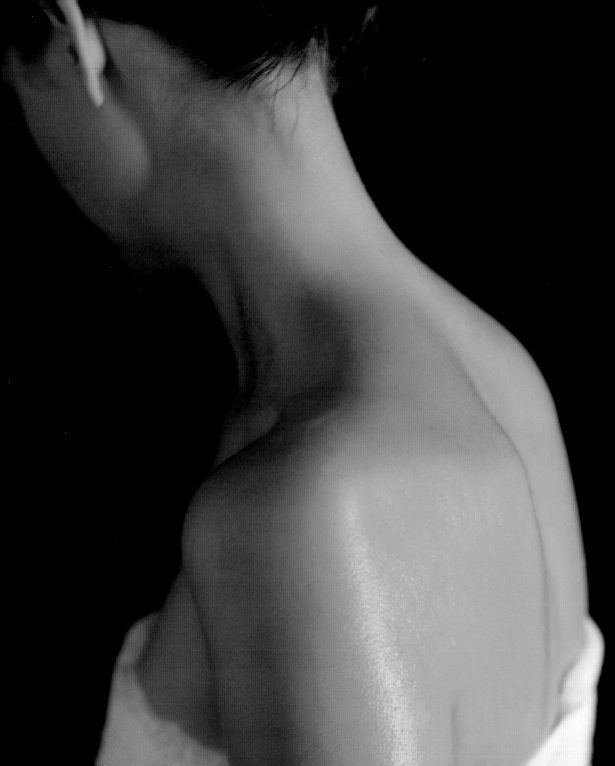

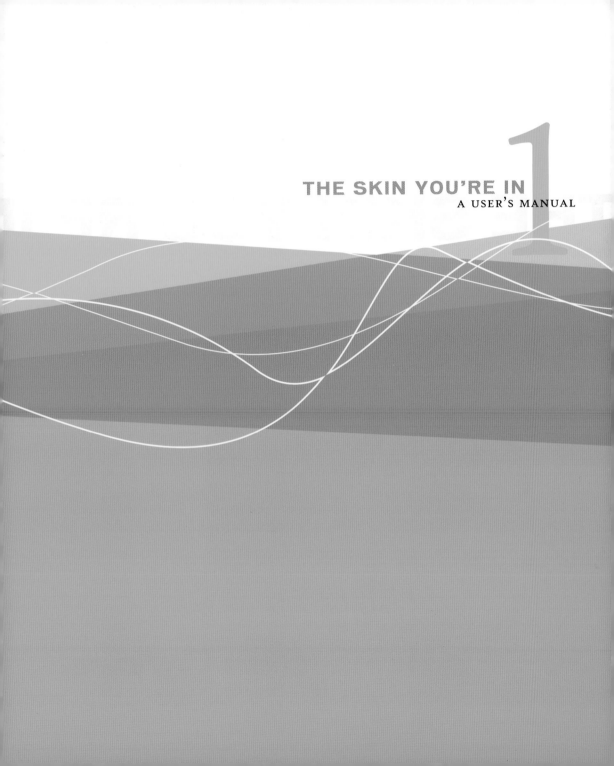

THE SKIN YOU'RE IN
A USER'S MANUAL

1

Your skin is more than just a cellophane wrapper. It is actually a vital organ that has the thankless job of blocking out the bad elements (bacteria and viruses, for example) and also of protecting and nourishing the body through temperature regulation, excretion of water and waste material, and absorption of vitamin D from sunlight.

None of this really comes to mind, however, when you wake up one morning and find a constellation of blemishes on your chin. The human body is a giant communications system, and nowhere is this more apparent than in the skin. This is why traditional Chinese doctors use the skin as a diagnostic tool; it is connected to all the systems of the body and can indicate the status of the circulatory, immune, digestive, and nervous systems. Whether you have raging PMS, are eating poorly, or are feeling stressed, your skin will tell the story.

A CROSS-SECTION OF THE SKIN

The skin has its own ecosystem that depends on a complex series of chemical processes. In this cycle, plump, new layers of cells, rich with the protein collagen, are built. These cells flatten out as they move toward the surface, and they are discarded when they reach the uppermost layer of skin, the EPI-DERMIS, every fourteen to twenty-eight days.

Below this layer lies the DERMIS, home to two critical types of connective tissue, collagen and elastin, responsible for the strength and elasticity of the skin. Nerve endings, hair follicles, and sweat glands are all embedded in the dermis. A network of thin blood vessels, called capillaries, helps move nutrients to the uppermost layer of the dermis and remove by-products of cellular waste.

The SUBCUTANEOUS LAYER, the deepest layer of the skin, provides support for veins and internal organs and is made of fat cells that help the body retain heat. Here, new skin cells are formed from nutrients carried by the capillaries.

Your skin is a vibrant organ that interacts with both internal and external forces on a daily basis as it seeks to maintain balance. To protect this complex organ and thereby prevent premature aging and other imbalances, you need to be an active participant in your overall health.

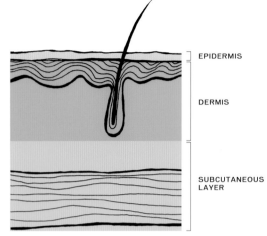

EPIDERMIS

DERMIS

SUBCUTANEOUS
LAYER

SKIN 101

Why is it that some of us seem to grow old gracefully while others watch our crow's-feet deepen and our forehead and chin turn into the Great Barrier Reef? We can blame this on a combination of our genes, our lifestyles, and our beauty regimens.

As we age, and beginning in our late thirties and forties, collagen and elastin, the structural proteins that give the skin support and elasticity, begin to break down. One explanation for the change is offered in the free-radical theory. Free radicals are not political activists; they're oxygen molecules that can bear free electrons. They are highly reactive and can weaken proteins when the body becomes vulnerable. As a result, the skin cells grow rigid as nutrients are locked out and wastes kept in, leading to wrinkled skin. With overexposure to external environmental aggressors such as the sun and pollution, and internal factors such as a poor diet and chronic lack of proper hydration, signs of aging gradually begin to creep up.

The role of glucose in the aging process has been popularized by Dr. Nicholas Perricone in his book *The Wrinkle Cure*. When high levels of glucose are present, irreversible cross-links between adjacent proteins are formed, contributing to a loss of elasticity in the skin. Eating low-glycemic (low sugar forming) foods goes a long way toward preventing this effect. See chapter 3 for more about glucose and its effects.

THE BEAUTY BASICS: TEN EASY STEPS

The essence of holistic skin care is simplicity. Having good skin does not mean keeping your medicine cabinet packed with a vast assortment of bottles and jars containing ingredients with seven syllables in their names. What your skin really wants is a dose of common sense and TLC, not product overload and complicated beauty regimens. For most of us, this might be as simple as using the correct cleanser or applying a vitamin-rich avocado oil at night.

STEP 1: CLEANSE, DON'T STRIP

Cleansing, the most important step in your beauty ritual, lays the proper foundation for correcting or fortifying your skin. The purpose of cleansing is to remove dirt and oil, both of which can block pores and lead to breakouts. Cleansers are made up of three main ingredients: a surfactant or wetting agent to reduce surface tension on the skin, oil to help to dissolve grease, and water to wash away dirt and grime. In order to clean the skin, a cleanser has to break down the hydrolipid barrier of the skin, the delicate layer of surface lipids made up of oil and water.

Unfortunately, this is not as easy as it sounds. A good cleanser will not strip away the beneficial oils of the skin along with the grime. Nor will it alter the slight level of acidity that is normally found in the skin and acts as a barrier to keep out bacteria. This is why you should never use soap, even handmade soap, on your face. Its alkalinity will upset the pH balance, cause irritation, and leave the skin feeling taut.

When choosing a cleanser, avoid those containing drying and irritating surfactants such as sodium lauryl sulfate (SLS) or sodium laureth sulfate. These surfactants have strong foaming properties that we've been taught to associate with clean skin, are sensitizing to the skin, cause comedones (blackheads), and can be irritating to the eyes. Choose instead a natural cleanser that uses coconut-derived fatty acids as surfactants, which won't create as much lather but will remove dirt and debris without causing irritation.

Most cleansers will dissolve water-based makeup, but for heavy, oil-based makeup use an all-natural baby wipe, sold in health food stores. These are free

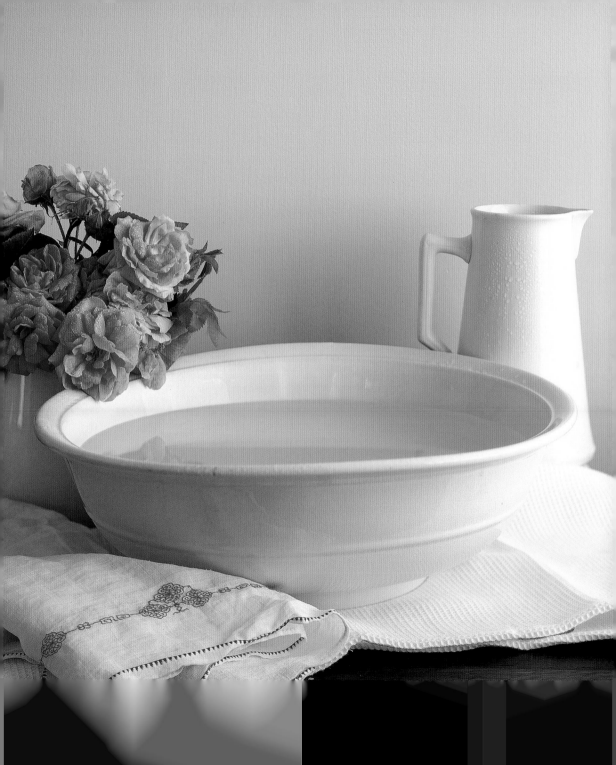

wash your face—
don't power wash it

AVOID OVERWASHING YOUR SKIN;
allow your face to maintain an ade-
quate amount of oil. People with dry
skin may only need to cleanse their
skin once a day; those with oily skin
should cleanse twice a day, but no
more.

BEGIN BY SPLASHING WARM (never
hot) WATER on your face to stimulate
blood circulation to the area.

APPLY A PEA-SIZED AMOUNT OF
CLEANSER to your fingertips and gently
work into the skin. Avoid using a washcloth or scrub pad on sensitive skin.

RINSE WITH COOL (not cold) WATER
to refresh the skin. The cooling action
will constrict the blood flow and trigger
a natural pumping action to remove
cellular waste material from the facial
tissues. Pat dry.

INVEST IN A GOOD WATER FILTER
for your shower. Chlorine is one of the
leading causes of dry skin, stripping the
skin of its protective hydrolipid barrier.
Furthermore, it can be toxic. See the resources section for water filter suppliers.

of irritating fragrance and propylene glycol and will easily remove
oil-based makeup. Wipe your skin gently.

After you cleanse, you'll want to tone your skin. The role
of toners is to correct the pH balance of the skin after cleansing
(although if you have chosen a proper cleanser your pH balance
won't need correcting). Contrary to popular belief, toners cannot make your pores smaller, because your pores do not open and
close. However, toners can deliver beneficial ingredients such as
essential oils to the skin. For example, floral waters, or hydrolats,
are a natural by-product of the distillation process of essential
oil. Hydrolats contain microscopic particles of plant material
suspended in water. Sprayed regularly onto the skin, these tiny
particles behave like homeopathic medicines, helping the skin
stay balanced.

STEP 2: SLOUGH

Exfoliation is the second most important step in skin care. Done regularly, it helps sweep away dirt and clear oil-clogged pores, both of
which can cause breakouts. An exfoliating scrub works by using a
physical agent such as jojoba beads to slough away dead skin. Avoid
facial scrubs that use ingredients like apricot seed or walnut shell as
exfoliating agents, since these will tear the delicate skin.

Using alpha hydroxy acids (AHAs) or glycolic acid is another
way to exfoliate the skin. AHAs are a group of naturally occurring
substances found in many common fruits and other foods; they
include citric acid from citrus fruit, malic acid from apples, tartaric
acid from grapes, and lactic acid from sour milk. Glycolic acid is
naturally derived from sugarcane.

AHAs and glycolic acid work by breaking down the protein
bonds making up the uppermost layer of the skin. By loosening
up the outer layer of skin, these acids cause a gentle exfoliation
of dry, dead skin cells and create a softer, smoother texture. Dermatologists consider glycolic acid to be particularly effective in
helping acne-prone skin, by dissolving the built-up dead cells in
the follicle.

Several of the leading natural skin care companies do not use AHAs or glycolics in their product lines because they feel that this exfoliation is not a "natural" process internally generated by the body. To be perfectly honest, I have never understood this controversy, since this is how most natural therapies work, by provoking a type of mild inflammatory response to induce a therapeutic reaction. For example, juniper oil, a natural diuretic, works by slightly irritating the kidneys.

Glycolics come in many different strengths, ranging from 5 percent (over the counter) to 30 percent (used in a dermatologist's office). However, it is not the strength of the glycolic but the pH level that makes them effective at softening the skin. Generally, the lower the pH level, the stronger the glycolic, and the deeper the exfoliating benefits.

STEP 3: FORTIFY

All skin is thirsty. Skin craves moisture, as well as vitamins and antioxidants, to protect it from internal free-radical damage and external environmental factors. A poor or damaging cleansing and toning program can dehydrate the skin.

One way you can fortify and protect your skin is by using either a face oil or serum. Although it might seem counterintuitive, there is absolutely nothing wrong with putting these high-quality oils on your face (yes, even if you have an oily complexion); they do not cause acne. Because oils have a small molecular structure, they are more easily absorbed into the skin than creams.

Unfortunately, many commercial face oils or serums contain base oils that have been extracted using a synthetic solvent such as hexane. Residue from hexane irritates the skin and can cause breakouts and rashes. Cold-pressed vegetal and nut oils are a healthier alternative. Since these oils are not heated extensively during the extraction process, they contain more of the healthy vitamins and nutrients that feed the skin.

Moisturizing lotions, creams, and balms contain an emulsion of water and oil that helps hold moisture in the skin and acts as a barrier to prevent water loss. In addition, moisturizers help fill in the gaps between skin cells caused by overstripping. Choose a moisturizer according to the amount of oil in your skin (an oily complexion will want a more fluid lotion while dry skin will need a heavier cream or balm). Keep in mind that, depending upon the season or climate, your skin will need more or less hydration at different times. Apply

holistic facial Rx

What sets a holistic facial apart from a standard deep-cleansing facial is the stimulation of the body's own natural healing systems, and the treatment of the cause of an imbalance rather than the symptom. Here is what to expect from a holistic facial, in addition to the standard cleansing, extraction, and hydration:

CONSULTATION AND ANALYSIS: Expect the esthetician to ask you about your needs and goals for the session and to analyze your skin. She'll also try to identify the mental, emotional, and lifestyle factors that may be influencing your skin.

LYMPHATIC STIMULATION: The lymphatic system is part of the body's immune and waste disposal system and consists of a network of fluid-filled vessels distributed throughout the body under the surface of the skin. During the session the esthetician will use lymphatic massage techniques to mechanically stimulate the flow of lymph, applying very light pressure on the surface of the skin.

MASSAGE STIMULATION: Firm, therapeutic massage brings blood, oxygen, and nutrients to the tissues and produces a gentle cleansing effect by removing cellular waste. A good treatment should not only include a stimulating facial massage but also a vigorous neck and shoulder massage to relax the entire body, which is equally important to the healing response.

EDUCATION: Your esthetician will teach you how to keep your skin looking radiant on a daily basis.

moisturizer after a bath or shower while the skin is still damp or mist your face with a floral water, or hydrolat, to increase water permeability.

STEP 4: SUN SURVIVAL

The facts: there is no such thing as a safe tan. Tanning is just as harmful as a burn. Some sunlight is essential for both our physical and emotional well-being, but excessive exposure to the sun causes the skin's collagen to break down, immediately prompting an inflammatory response in the body. It also causes wrinkles and dark spots, and it gives the skin a leathery texture as the skin tries to build up a thicker outer layer to protect the body.

Be smart: make putting on sunblock a part of your daily regimen today. Only a natural, full-spectrum sunblock such as titanium dioxide or zinc oxide will block out both UVA and UVB, because it acts as a physical barrier on the skin to reflect these harmful rays. You may find that these sunblocks are harder to rub in than chemical-based sunblocks like Octyl Methoxycinnamate or Parasol, but be patient. The benefits are worth the extra effort because synthetic sunblocks are loaded with skin-irritating ingredients. Make sure you apply enough sunblock to cover the exposed areas— use 1 ounce (enough to fill a shot glass) for the entire body, and reapply every 2 hours. And don't forget to protect your eyes: wear sunglasses with 98-percent UV protection.

STEP 5: PUT YOUR BEST FACE FORWARD

While in the past spas were a place for a day of luxurious rest and relaxation, today top spas focus less on pampering and more on teaching clients about health and well-being with results-oriented treatments. These skin-care centers employ top estheticians (and sometimes even dermatologists) to get your skin looking its best.

Find a good spa in your area and have a facial at the very least four times a year, with the change of the seasons. A good facial goes a long way toward flawless skin. An esthetician can give you a deeper cleansing and exfoliation than you can give yourself at home; however, at-home facials are an option as well.

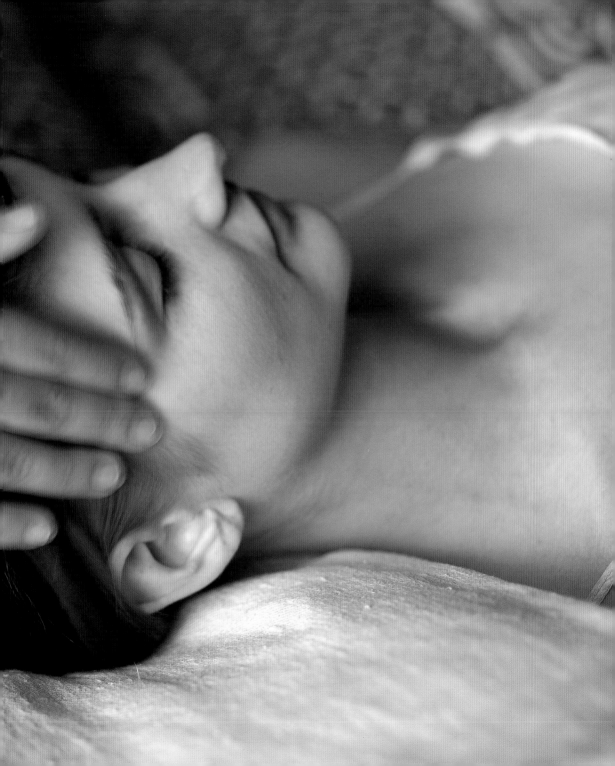

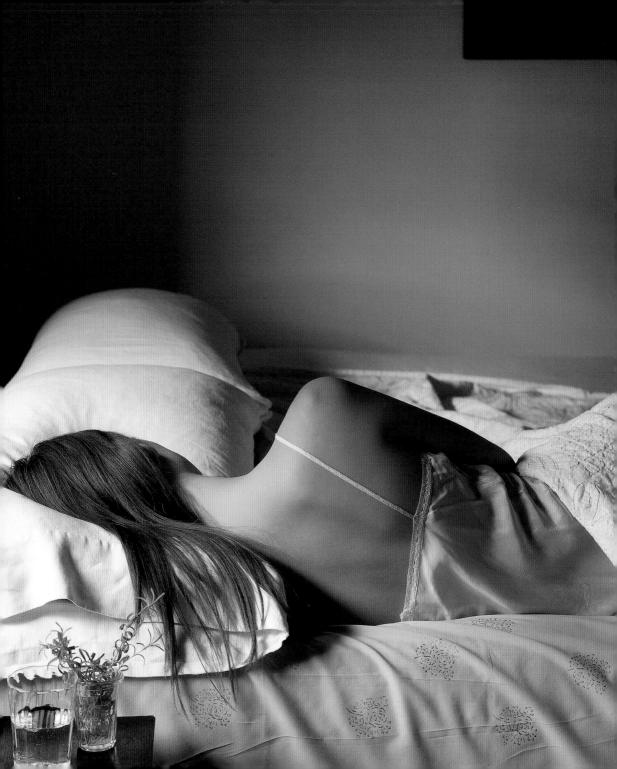

There are some essentials you need to look for in a good facial. You want high-quality, clean, natural products that support the integrity of the skin. A good facial will also address the main cleansing systems of the body, the lymphatic and circulatory system.

STEP 6: SLEEP

They don't call it beauty sleep for nothing. Make sure you get at least seven to eight hours of sleep most nights. This allows your mind and body, including your skin, time to rest and regenerate, right down to the cellular level.

STEP 7: CLIMATE CONTROL

Sahara-like air caused by central heating and air-conditioning systems steals moisture from your skin on a daily basis. While it may not be possible to move to a tropical island to give your skin that moisture it craves, there are steps you can take to minimize water loss from the skin. Invest in a humidifier for your bedroom so that the humectants in your moisturizer don't have to work as hard to pull moisture into your skin's ecosystem (see Resources, page 142).

To supplement this nighttime regimen, get in the habit of carrying a bottle of floral water, or hydrolat, in your purse. Liberally mist your skin throughout the day. Not only will this help prevent water loss but the aromatic essences will refresh you as well. This is an absolute must for airplane travel.

STEP 8: EVERYTHING IN MODERATION– EVEN MODERATION

Cigarette packs in Europe carry the following warning statement: "Smoking kills. Stopping smoking reduces the risk of fatal heart and lung diseases." Smoking is horrible for the skin as well and causes premature aging much like the sun does. Try to kick the habit. If you must smoke, switch to organic tobacco.

As for other vices, I am the last person who would to discourage you from having a glass of good wine. But remember that drinking alcohol dehydrates the skin and can cause broken capillaries

quick tips to help you sleep

MAKE LUNCH, NOT DINNER, YOUR BIGGEST MEAL OF THE DAY. Eat foods such as salmon and turkey that are fortified with tryptophan, an amino acid that causes production of the sleep-inducing chemicals serotonin and melatonin.

EXERCISE REGULARLY. This helps control cortisol levels, helping you sleep.

AVOID AFTERNOON NAPS longer than twenty minutes.

AVOID ALCOHOL and NICOTINE before bed.

Develop a REGULAR BEDTIME ROUTINE.

DRINK A CUP OF RELAXING HERBAL TEA or TAKE A BATH to help yourself wind down an hour before bedtime.

CREATE AN ENVIRONMENT THAT IS CONDUCIVE TO SLEEP–make your bedroom a dark, comfortable haven.

USE SCENT TO INDUCE SLUMBER: Place 3 or 4 drops of a calming essential oil like lavender or vanilla on a tissue and slide it underneath the pillowcase or add the oil to a diffuser lamp.

Before bed give yourself, or exchange with a partner, a relaxing FOOT MASSAGE (see page 92).

when consumed in excess. Try to stick to beer and wine and avoid hard liquor. Offset alcohol intake with lots of water: FOR EVERY GLASS OF ALCOHOL CONSUMED, YOU NEED TO DRINK TWO GLASSES OF WATER. And on those nights when you've lost all control, drink a liter of water before your head hits the pillow.

STEP 9: WORK IT OUT

Exercise does more for your skin than any skin-care cream will and is second only to diet in maintaining healthy skin. Exercise gives your body a surge of oxygen to all the organs, and the skin is a major beneficiary of this process, since oxygen enables it to work more efficiently. Increased oxygen intake, especially during exercise, prevents free-radical damage, a causative factor in premature aging of the skin. Working out promotes the cleansing of the blood by stimulating circulation and perspiration, which aid the skin's metabolism as well.

Researchers now believe that even small amounts of exercise, such as 30 minutes per day, can yield positive benefits. Begin by making small changes in your daily routine—use the stairs instead of riding the elevator, walk during your lunch hour, park your car at the far end of the lot when you go to the shopping mall—that will help to keep your complexion rosy and your jeans comfortable. For a more intense oxygen cleansing of the lungs and skin, try an aerobic activity such as running, swimming, or biking. Yoga is also a highly beneficial activity, because deep stretching releases toxins in the spine and joints and deep breathing brings oxygen to the body.

STEP 10: THE STRESSLESS STEP

You find yourself racing toward home while inhaling a slice of pizza behind the wheel or arguing with your mother-in-law on the phone at work while analyzing a spreadsheet before a critical meeting. Stress-free? You must be joking.

Prolonged stress causes the release of the hormone cortisol in the body, which is a major contributor to numerous health problems, including reduced immunity, heart disease, digestive upset, chronic pain, sexual dysfunction, insomnia, or depression. The skin, interacting with the circulatory, nervous, and immune system, as well as reacting to your emotional swings, often manifests its own set of problems, such as acne, eczema, hives, psoriasis, and rosacea. Try to keep your stress level within healthy limits to avoid imbalances.

beauty dopp kit

During World War II, recruits were issued travel kits, called "Dopp kits," that contained all standard-issue and emergency gear that a soldier carried on a regular basis.

In order to achieve healthy skin, focusing on inner beauty and not just topical treatments, you will need to stock up on the essentials listed below to create your own beauty Dopp Kit. The specific properties of each of these remedies are outlined in further detail in chapters that follow.

THE GREEN ROUTINE

Purchase skin-friendly, chemical-free beauty essentials: SULFATE-FREE CLEANSER, EXFOLIANT, HYDROLAT TONER, FACE OIL, MOISTURIZER, EYE CREAM, and SUNBLOCK. These basics will go a long way toward helping you to look your best.

HERBAL REMEDIES

Herbs contain many highly active ingredients and balancing secondary ingredients that work synergistically to make them a potent form of natural medicine. Herbal medicines use these therapeutic properties to support the body's self-healing powers. The following skin-clarifying herbs are potent allies, helping the skin function optimally: DANDELION ROOT, MILK THISTLE, ECHINACEA, RED CLOVER, BURDOCK ROOT, STINGING NETTLE, YELLOW DOCK, PSYLLIUM HUSK, and GREEN TEA EXTRACT. Taken singly or combined, these herbs can be ingested as a liquid extract or in capsule form.

BEAUTY VITAMINS AND SUPPLEMENTS

Forget what the health stores claim; you don't need to take a fistful of vitamins every day. Good health comes from good food. However, taking a good multivitamin goes a long way toward ensuring that your skin has the vitamins and essential fatty acids it needs. Vitamin A is essential for normal development of skin and other epithelial tissues, B-complex vitamins help bring blood to the tissues and vitamin C is a powerful antioxidant.

If you are traveling and you don't have your multivitamins with you, drink vitamin-fortified water or add an effervescent vitamin packet to water or juice.

HOMEOPATHIC REMEDIES

Homeopathy, developed in the late 1700s, is based on the principle that like cures like. In this system of medicine, an illness is treated by the administration of minute doses of a natural substance that would cause symptoms similar to those of the illness if administered in high doses. The body is then able to gently heal itself by working against that substance.

The following homeopathic remedies are useful in treating skin imbalances and stress-related conditions: CALCAREA SULPHURICA, NATRUM MURIATICUM, ARNICA MONTANA, and COFFEA CRUDA.

FLOWER ESSENCES

During the 1930s, Dr. Edward Bach discovered the thirty-eight flower essences. These homeopathic remedies represent a complete system of healing that focuses on the personality, mood, and emotional outlook of an individual.

Since stress is at the root of many skin imbalances, make sure to include flower essences in your beauty Dopp Kit to soothe emotional upsets. Include RESCUE REMEDY (see page 140) or try a custom blend of remedies that would work best for your particular needs.

AROMATHERAPY

Aromatherapy is the art and science of using volatile essential oils of plants—often referred to as a plant's "life force"—for healing. Genuine essential oils—not synthetic fragrances—can assist in the maintenance of healthy skin and body, from treating blemishes and rashes to keeping your moods balanced.

Use TEA TREE OIL to treat blemishes. Place 3 drops of MANDARIN OIL on a tissue and put it under your pillowcase to help you sleep.

ASSORTED ESSENTIALS

These are the extras you can't live without:

NATURAL BABY WIPES—to remove oil-based makeup

SLEEP MASK—for essential beauty sleep

HYDROLATS—for misting onto your face throughout the day to allow the concentrated plant extract to rebalance and fortify the skin (a must for air travel)

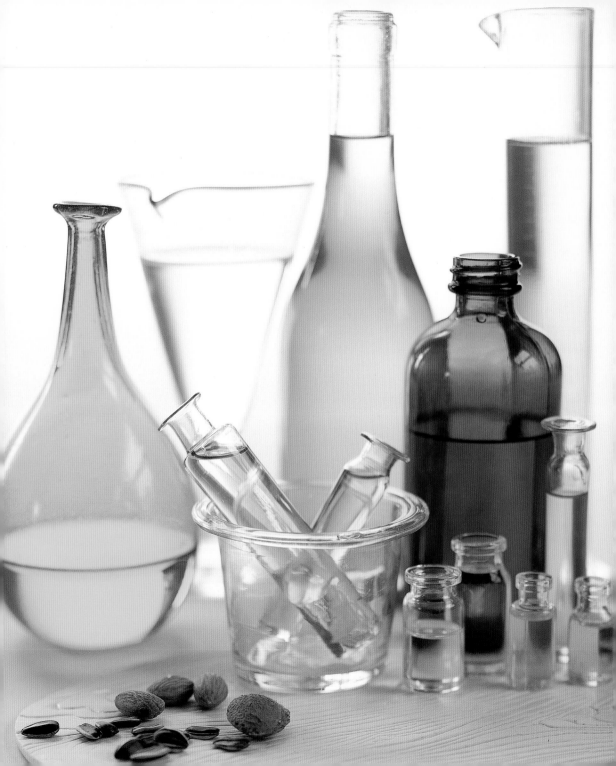

BEAUTY RITUALS
FOR YOUR SKIN PERSONALITY

(B) (HR) (SR) (ER) (M)

Every skin personality is unique and has its own recommended beauty rituals to achieve optimal performance. These next few pages will help you identify which of the five skin personalities is yours and provide the necessary step to help you care for your skin from the inside out. Don't worry if you are unfamiliar with some of the procedures or ingredients—all of the essentials will be covered in later chapters.

PERSONALITY

In the late 1960s, a trend toward "scientific" skin care led to the introduction of the three skin types that we know today: normal, dry, and oily. This classification system went on to dominate the skin-care industry and changed how women looked at their skin. Even today, your skin type is determined by how much or little oil your skin produces, using the usual classification system:

NORMAL: medium-sized pores, smooth skin tone
OILY: enlarged pores, shiny skin, prone to blemishes
DRY: small pores, tight skin tone, some flaking

The reasoning behind this classification system is that by knowing your skin type you can better understand how to minimize irritation and help to correct problems.

Skin typing, while a useful topical diagnostic tool, is overly simplistic and does not tell the whole story of how or why the skin has become imbalanced. Oily or dry skin is the result of a systemic imbalance within the body and begs the question, what are the causative factors that have given rise to this condition? The cause may have multiple origins affecting mind, body, and spirit. Until the cause has been addressed, the condition cannot be effectively treated.

A holistic approach to well-being and beauty always looks at symptoms from an in-depth perspective, since symptoms are simply messages that the body is sending us. I prefer to call my classifications "skin personalities" instead of skin types because I think this more accurately reflects how our bodies, and in particular our skin as a living, communicating organ, work. Skin personalities can be broken down into five main groups.

BALANCED

I have always disliked the skin-type label "normal," because it implies that everyone who does not fit that description is somehow inferior (are they "abnormal"?). A balanced skin personality is one in which the types of problems have a fairly narrow range and one that requires minimal attention. Over 75 percent of women fall into this category.

HORMONE REACTIVE

This personality is somewhat mercurial, its swings determined by the ebb and flow of hormones. This can be due to the normal course of a woman's menstrual cycle or the onset of menopause. The specific hormones that create havoc in the skin are androgens, which stimulate the sebum glands to enlarge and make more oil. As the sebum glands expand, the extra oil they secrete clogs the pores, causing acne. Hormone-reactive skin tends to have enlarged pores and excessive oiliness and is prone to acne-related conditions.

STRESS REACTIVE

Stress creates havoc in our bodies. It causes our adrenal glands to work overtime, producing excessive amounts of corticoids that not only raise our "fight or flight" response but also create problems for the endocrine system. Decreased immune resistance, circulatory problems such as high blood pressure, and skin imbalances such as blemishes, rosacea, dermatitis, eczema, and psoriasis are all exacerbated by stress. Stress-reactive skin has an average pore size and moderate oil production (mainly in the T zone) but is highly sensitive to lifestyle factors such as lack of sleep, poor diet, and a stressful schedule.

ENVIRONMENT REACTIVE

In addition to helping to monitor the internal environment of the body, the skin must also react to external forces that bear down upon it. Changes in temperature, sunlight, humidity, and allergens in the environment all have a direct effect on the clarity of the skin. Modern living really challenges the skin's ability to adapt—it has to deal with everything from overheated office buildings to decompressed airplanes and urban air quality. Environment reactive skin has an average pore size and moderate oil production but can display symptoms such as dermatitis, dry and flaky skin, and rashes due to changes in the environment.

MATURE

Despite the many antiaging treatments on the market, the truth is that time does the same thing to everyone: it ages the skin. Certainly there are factors that can hasten this process; overexposure to sunlight, smoking, and absence of proper skin care are some of them. The mature skin personality has a thinner epithelial layer, lacks moisture, and shows facial lines and wrinkles as well as sun damage.

BALANCED SKIN

B

SKIN-CARE REGIMEN

CLEANSING: Adjust cleansing regimen as needed, using a sulfate-free gel-based cleanser when skin is in oily phase and a cream cleanser during dry phase. Wash once, or, if necessary, twice a day. Look for toning herbs such as LAVENDER, ROSEMARY VERBENONE, ROMAN CHAMOMILE, and MEADOWSWEET to help balance the skin. Try the CLARIFYING CLEANSING OIL recipe on page 72.

EXFOLIATING: Use an alpha hydroxy acid or fruit enzyme peel two or three times a week or try the CLEANSING FACIAL GOMAGE on page 73.

TONING: Use ROMAN CHAMOMILE, LAVENDER, or MELISSA HYDROLAT after cleansing or exfoliating. Try the GREEN TEA TONER recipe on page 75.

MOISTURIZING: Use a lightweight face serum made from vegetal oils such as JOJOBA and APRICOT KERNEL with balancing essential oils such as NEROLI, ROMAN CHAMOMILE, and FRANKINCENSE. Or try the NEROLI TONING SERUM recipe on page 80.

Look for a light– to medium-weight moisturizer containing antioxidants such as VITAMINS A, C, and E and EVENING PRIMROSE OIL, rich in gamma linoleic acid (GLA), an essential fatty acid used in collagen production. Always apply sunblock to skin before going outdoors.

SKIN FITNESS

Eat the BEAUTY FOODS outlined on page 101 and follow the FOURTEEN-DAY DETOX PLAN on page 110 in spring and fall to cleanse and renew the body. Do the follow-up WEEKEND DETOX on page 111 as needed.

HERBAL REMEDY CHEST

HERBAL REMEDIES: Drink 5 cups of green tea daily.

Apply TEA TREE OIL directly onto skin with cotton swab to help clear up occasional breakouts.

FLOWER ESSENCES: Take appropriate FLOWER ESSENCE (see page 140) daily.

SKINCEUTICALS

Take a multivitamin daily.

Take extra doses of vitamin C during stressful periods to bolster the immune system and to support the collagen and elastin matrix of the skin.

BEAUTY AND BALANCE

Select a relaxing ritual to practice daily, such as gardening, knitting, or yoga.

Try to incorporate a monthly maintenance program of massage or heat therapy with sauna or steam.

SPECIAL RX

Boost skin with a reviving face mask once a week to brighten complexion.

Try the CLARIFYING FACIAL SAUNA on page 74.

Incorporate a facial massage with your choice of serum twice a month to stimulate circulation and give the skin a healthy glow (see page 84).

SKIN-CARE EXPRESS

Begin each day with a LAVENDER COMPRESS (see page 84) to boost circulation

Add an effervescent vitamin powder to water and drink to bolster the immune system during stressful periods.

Get a holistic deep-cleansing facial a minimum of four times a year.

HORMONE-REACTIVE SKIN

do any of the
following descriptions
apply to your skin?

◇ skin breaks out before
menstrual period

◇ skin was blemish-free
until your late forties

◇ blemishes tend to be
larger, deeper, and
cystlike, often appearing
on lower cheeks and chin

◇ skin is prone to oiliness

◇ enlarged pore size

SKIN-CARE REGIMEN

CLEANSING: Use a sulfate-free gel-based cleanser containing antiseptic herbs such as TEA TREE, CYPRESS or JUNIPER no more than twice a day to combat oiliness.

EXFOLIATING: Exfoliate daily with a glycolic solution containing salicylic acid to unclog pores or try the CLEANSING FACIAL GOMAGE recipe on page 73.

TONING: Use LAVENDER, NEROLI, or JUNIPER HYDROLAT or try the CLARIFYING PARSLEY TONER recipe on page 77.

MOISTURIZING: Use a lightweight face serum with a base of a slightly astringent vegetal oil such as HAZELNUT and combine with antiseptic essential oils such as LAVENDER, TEA TREE, and LEMON. Try the ROSEMARY ACNE SERUM on page 82.

Look for a lightweight or oil-reducing moisturizer with antioxidants such as vitamins A, C, and E. Make sure moisturizer does not have acne-exacerbating ingredients such as lanolin, mineral oil, and other petroleum-based products. Always apply sunblock to skin before going outdoors.

SKIN FITNESS

Eat the BEAUTY FOODS outlined on page 101 and enjoy plenty of foods containing vitamin B6, such as OILY FISH, YOGURT, EGGS, BANANAS, AVOCADO and CAULIFLOWER, which can help balance hormone levels. Avoid foods that contain iodides, such as shellfish, seaweed, and iodide salt, which can aggravate acne. Try to eat soy-based foods that contain phytoestrogens (i.e., plant estrogens). These can help to modulate the effects of estrogen, a causative factor in acne flare-ups. Do the FOURTEEN-DAY DETOX PLAN on page 110 in spring and fall to cleanse and renew the body. Do the follow-up WEEKEND DETOX on page 111 as needed.

HERBAL REMEDY CHEST

HERBAL REMEDIES: Take hormone-balancing herbs such as CHASTE TREE BERRY (also known as AGNUS-CASTUS) and DONG QUAI. (NOTE: Do not take dong quai during pregnancy.) These herbs can be ingested as herbal extracts and added to hot water, juice, or tea or taken in capsule form. Drink the COMPLEXION TEA on page 137. Apply TEA TREE ESSENTIAL OIL or MOSS EXTRACT directly onto skin with a cotton swab to help clear up breakouts.

FLOWER ESSENCES: Take appropriate FLOWER ESSENCE (see page 140) daily.

HOMEOPATHIC REMEDY: Try PULSATILLA PRATENSIS, a useful remedy for individuals who are prone to emotional swings and find that skin tends to worsen during these periods.

continued

SPECIAL RX

Do not overwash skin. This causes oil glands to overcompensate and produce more oil.

Do not pop pimples. But since you are going to do this anyway, here's how: gently squeeze pimple with clean hands wrapped in cotton or tissues. Sweep away debris and dab with tea tree oil. Do not touch!

Make the PURIFYING GREEN TEA MASK (page 86) and leave on for 10 minutes to kill the bacteria that cause blemishes.

SKIN-CARE EXPRESS

Mist face with antiseptic hydrolat or toner throughout the day to keep skin free of bacteria.

Schedule monthly facials to help control acne flare-ups.

SKINCEUTICALS
Take a multivitamin daily.

Take an additional 250 milligrams of a vitamin A, which can help reduce sebum production. (NOTE: Pregnant women should not take large doses vitamin A, which can cause birth defects.)

BEAUTY AND BALANCE
Since hormone-reactive skin can be stressful to live with, be sure to incorporate some stress-reducing activities such as walking, meditation, and hearty laughter into your daily routine.

Schedule a weekly WATER CURE (see page 127): try a relaxing herbal bath featuring CLARY SAGE, an herb possessing estrogen-like qualities and used to ease premenstrual symptoms.

The feet have hundreds of nerve endings and can benefit from daily foot massages to relax overstimulated nerve pathways and reduce hormonal swings. Try the easy FOOT MASSAGE on page 92.

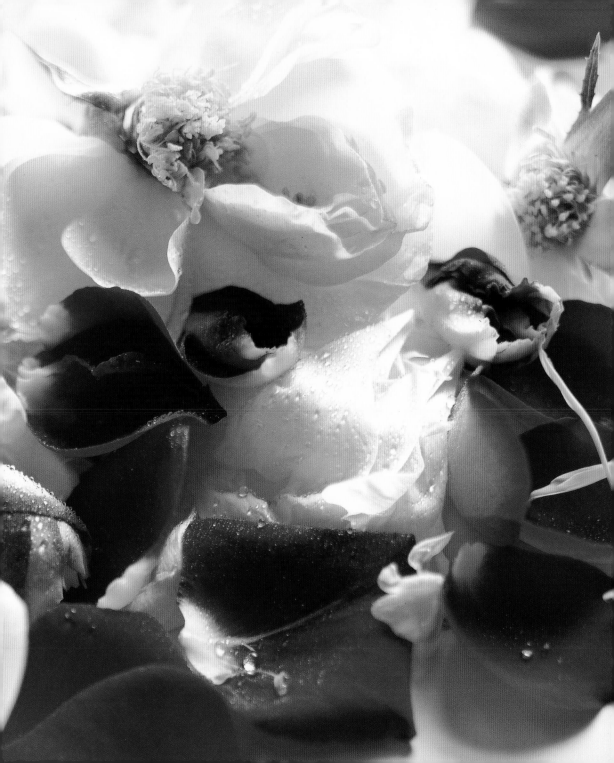

STRESS-REACTIVE SKIN

do any of the
following descriptions
apply to your skin?

◇ skin breaks out during
stressful periods

◇ blemishes are small,
usually located around
mouth and chin area

◇ skin produces moderate
oil, mostly in T zone area

◇ episodes of red, rashy
skin or flaky patches of
dry skin, especially
on face, hands, feet,
or elbows

◇ family history of psoriasis,
eczema, hives, or other
skin imbalances

SKIN-CARE REGIMEN

CLEANSING: Once a day use a soothing sulfate-free cleansing cream containing an anti-inflammatory herb such as GERMAN CHAMOMILE, ALOE, or ROSE. Or make your own CLEANSING FACIAL GOMAGE (see page 73).

EXFOLIATING: Do not exfoliate skin during reactive phases, when rash or itching is present. During dormant phases, exfoliate the skin with a fruit enzyme such as PAPAYA or PUMPKIN or use the CLEANSING FACIAL GOMAGE on page 73 daily.

TONING: Calm irritated skin with a rose hydrolat or try the PLANT MILK recipe on page 78.

MOISTURIZING: Use medium-weight face serum with a base of vegetal oil such as AVOCADO, rich in nutrients and beneficial for cell regeneration. Look for a skin-soothing essential oil such as CARROT SEED, ROSE, or GERMAN CHAMOMILE to add to the base oil. Try the CARROT SEED PROTECTIVE SERUM on page 81.

Look for a rich moisturizer containing skin-calming ingredients such as OAT BETA GLUCAN (derived from oatmeal), STINGING NETTLE, and SEA ALGAE EXTRACT as well as antioxidants such as vitamins A, C, and E. Always apply sunblock to skin before going outdoors.

SKIN FITNESS

Eat the BEAUTY FOODS outlined on page 101. Watch out for sugar and high-glycemic foods that cause an inflammatory response in the body (see page 100), especially since you may be more attracted to these during stressful periods. Avoid spicy foods as well as dairy products, since they may help to create heat in the skin thus aggravating skin imbalances. Do the FOURTEEN-DAY DETOX PLAN on page 110 twice a year to cleanse the system of the residue from stress-related eating. If skin becomes red, scaly, and itchy for a prolonged phase, take a pH test.

HERBAL REMEDY CHEST

AROMATHERAPY: Place a few drops of a calming essential oil such as LAVENDER, LEMON VERBENA, or CLARY SAGE in a diffuser lamp or on the pulse points on the inside of your wrists to help rebalance the mind and body throughout the day.

HERBAL REMEDIES: Take skin-clarifying herbs such as RED CLOVER, BURDOCK, YELLOW DOCK, STINGING NETTLE, MILK THISTLE, and DANDELION, which cleanse the blood and help the liver remove toxins more efficiently. For daily maintenance, take an energizing herb such as GINSENG to help strengthen the body and to support overtaxed adrenal glands. To help calm overstimulated nerves that have become frayed from severe itching, try a sedative herb such as SKULLCAP or VALERIAN. All of these herbs can be ingested as herbal extracts and added to hot water, juice, or tea or taken in capsule form (see pages 132-133).

FLOWER ESSENCES: Take appropriate FLOWER ESSENCE daily and use RESCUE REMEDY, a blend of anxiety-reducing flower essences, during high-stress periods (see page 140).

continued

SPECIAL RX

Avoid hot showers and baths when skin is irritated. Try to bathe once a day in cool water and as quickly as possible so as not to strip the body of precious oil. Apply a thick moisturizing cream immediately after patting yourself dry.

Look for skin-soothers in creams or balms, such as ALOE VERA GEL, CALENDULA, OATMEAL, and BURDOCK, to calm irritated skin. Try the HEALING CALENDULA SALVE recipe on page 134.

Sleep is the best antidote for skin problems caused by stress. Don't let anything interfere with your getting the minimum of eight hours your body needs. Stick to a regular sleep schedule during stressful times. Read the sleep tips on page 21.

If your skin becomes irritated frequently, buy a pH test kit at your drug store to determine the acidity of your body. If your level of acidity is too high, avoid acid-forming

continued

foods, which create skin disturbances such as rashes, hives, and
intense itching (see page 101).

SKIN-CARE EXPRESS

Fortify your skin with extra omega-3
fatty acids during especially stressful
times—eat salmon or other oily fish
and sprinkle flaxseed on salads.

During times of acute skin irritation, try the SOOTHING BURDOCK SOUP
on page 138.

Mist face with a calming hydrolat or
PLANT MILK (see page 78) throughout
the day (try keeping hydrolat in the
refrigerator for added cooling and
calming action).

Make a LAVENDER COMPRESS (see page
84) and apply to face as needed to
soothe irritated skin.

Get a holistic deep-cleansing facial
four times a year and book a professional massage once a month during
stressful periods.

HOMEOPATHIC REMEDIES: If you tend to worry compulsively,
try ARSENICUM ALBUM. During skin flare-ups, take CALCAREA
SULPHURICA to calm down irritated skin.

SKINCEUTICALS
Take a multivitamin daily.

Take 500 milligrams of BLACK CURRANT OIL twice a day to calm
down dry, red, irritated skin. Black currant oil contains gamma
linoleic acid (GLA), an omega-6 fatty acid that promotes healthy
growth of skin. You should begin to notice positive changes in
six to eight weeks.

BEAUTY AND BALANCE
Accept that some stress-related skin problems may be out of your
control. Try to incorporate some of the stress-balancing techniques outlined in chapter 4 such as the REST HERBAL BATH (see
page 128).

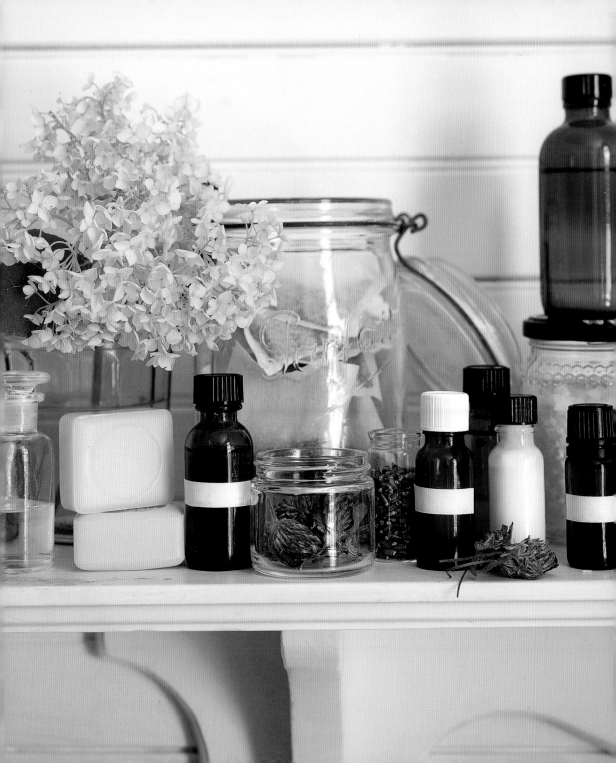

ENVIRONMENT-REACTIVE SKIN

do any of the
following descriptions
apply to your skin?

◇ skin breaks out with
change of seasons,
temperature, or humidity

◇ episodes of red, rashy
skin or flaky patches of
dry skin especially
on face, hands, feet,
or elbows

◇ hivelike skin rashes
appear when you use
skin and body care
products with particular
fragrances added, or
when you're exposed to
household detergents
or cleaning agents

◇ dark circles underneath
the eyes

◇ periodic allergy attacks

◇ moderate oil production

SKIN-CARE REGIMEN

CLEANSING: Once a day, use a soothing fragrance- and sulfate-free cream cleanser with anti-inflammatory herbs such as ALOE and ROSE. Or, make your own CLEANSING FACIAL GOMAGE (see page 73).

EXFOLIATING: Avoid glycolic and fruit enzymes that can exacerbate skin irritation.

TONING: Calm irritated skin by using a ROSE hydrolat or PLANT MILK (see page 78).

MOISTURIZING: Use medium-weight face serum with a base of vegetal oil such as AVOCADO or ROSE HIP. Try the CARROT SEED PROTECTIVE SERUM on page 81.

Look for a rich moisturizer containing skin-calming ingredients such as CALENDULA, BURDOCK, and SEA ALGAE EXTRACT as well as antioxidants such as vitamins A, C, and E. Avoid all creams with artificial fragrances as well as those containing urea or paraben preservatives. Always apply sunblock to skin before going outdoors.

SKIN FITNESS

Eat the BEAUTY FOODS outlined on page 101. Avoid sugar and high-glycemic foods that cause an inflammatory response in the body (see page 100) and stick to a diet rich in antioxidant foods. If skin becomes red, scaly, and itchy for a prolonged phase, create a food journal (see page 101) to identify a specific allergen, such as WHEAT, SOY, or CORN, which may be the culprit. Do the FOURTEEN-DAY DETOX PLAN on page 110 in the spring and fall and do the follow-up WEEKEND DETOX on page 111 as needed.

HERBAL REMEDY CHEST

HERBAL REMEDIES: Take skin-clarifying herbs such as RED CLOVER, BURDOCK, YELLOW DOCK, STINGING NETTLE, MILK THISTLE, and DANDELION, which cleanse the blood and help the liver remove toxins more efficiently. To help calm over-stimulated nerves that have become frayed from severe itching, try a sedative herb such as SKULLCAP or VALERIAN. All of these herbs can be ingested as herbal extracts and added to hot water, juice, or tea or taken in capsule form.

Look for creams and balms containing skin-soothing herbs such as ALOE VERA GEL, CHAMOMILE, CALENDULA, ST. JOHN'S WORT, and CARROT SEED to calm irritated skin. Try the HEALING CALENDULA SALVE recipe on page 134.

FLOWER ESSENCES: Take appropriate FLOWER ESSENCE (see page 140) daily.

HOMEOPATHIC REMEDY: NATRUM MURIATICUM is a good homeopathic remedy for sensitivity to the environment or allergies in general. SULPHUR is also an excellent homeopathic remedy for skin that is dry, itchy, and irritated as a result of bathing.

continued

SPECIAL RX

Clean out your medicine cabinet: throw away all skin-care products that contain potentially irritating ingredients (see list on page 47).

Purchase a neti pot, also called a nasal irrigation vessel, from a health food store. Fill with warm water and add 1 drop of TEA TREE OIL or 1/2 teaspoon SEA SALT. Irrigate sinuses once a day.

Rid your home of environmental pollutants: use organic cotton bed sheets, install an air purifier, change showerhead to a filtered attachment, use filtered water for cooking and drinking, and use environmentally friendly household cleaning products (see resources on page 142).

Buy a humidifier for your bedroom to let your skin recharge with eight hours of moisture every night. Be sure to clean the filter regularly and add a calming essential oil to the water to help you relax.

continued

Avoid products containing alpha hydroxy acids (AHA) and beta hydroxy acids (BHA), which can cause additional irritation to skin.

SKIN-CARE EXPRESS

Fortify your skin with extra OMEGA-3 FATTY ACIDS during especially stressful times—eat salmon or other oily fish and sprinkle FLAXSEED on salads.

During times of acute skin irritation, try the SOOTHING BURDOCK SOUP on page 138.

Mist face with calming hydrolat or PLANT MILK (see page 78) throughout the day (try keeping hydrolat in the refrigerator for added cooling and calming action).

Make a LAVENDER COMPRESS (see page 84) and apply to face as needed to soothe irritated skin.

SKINCEUTICALS

Take a multivitamin daily.

Take 500 milligrams of BLACK CURRANT OIL twice a day to soothe dry, irritated skin. Black currant oil contains gamma linoleic aid (GLA), an omega-6 fatty acid that promotes healthy growth of skin. You should begin to notice positive changes in six to eight weeks.

BEAUTY AND BALANCE

Enjoy a yoga class two or three times a week. Try visualization techniques to help decompress or, upon waking, try sitting and meditating for 15 to 20 minutes before rising for the day.

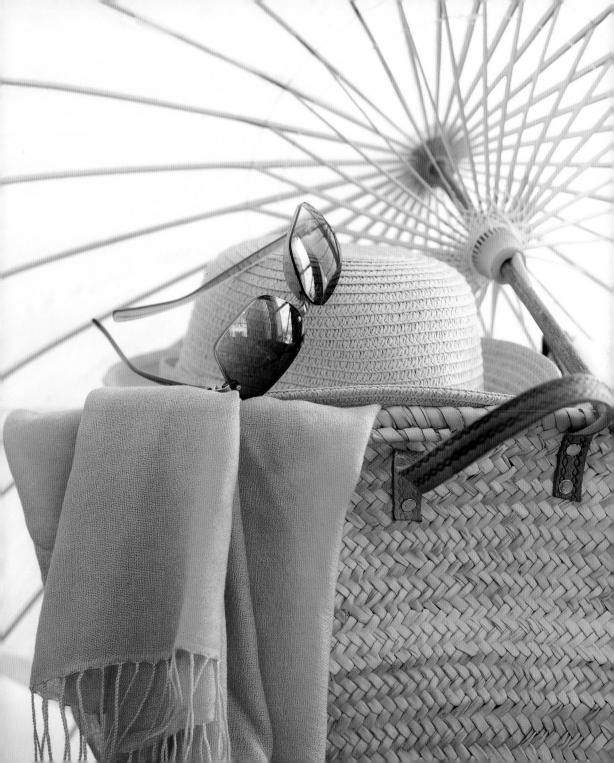

MATURE SKIN

do any of the
following descriptions
apply to your skin?

◇ skin shows wrinkles, dark
spots, or discoloration

◇ epidermis feels thinner
and drier than it used to

◇ skin produces little oil

◇ skin is not as firm as it
once was

◇ broken capillaries appear
especially on nose and
cheeks

SKIN-CARE REGIMEN

CLEANSING: Once a day, use a rich sulfate-free cream cleanser with hydrating plant extracts such as ALOE, GERMAN CHAMOMILE, and OATMEAL. Or make your own CLEANSING FACIAL GOMAGE (see page 73). Once a month, have a holistic deep-cleansing and hydrating facial.

EXFOLIATING: Exfoliate several times a week using a mask or gel; choose either an enzyme peel with ingredients such as BLACK CHERRY, RED WINE or PUMPKIN, or a SUGARCANE-DERIVED GLYCOLIC ACID. (Unless your skin is sensitive, look for a product with 10 percent glycolic acid and a pH level of less than 3, as this is what will break down the proteins of the skin. A higher pH will not be as effective.)

TONING: Use rose hydrolat or try the PLANT MILK on page 78.

MOISTURIZING: Use heavy-weight face serum with a blend composed of rich vegetal oils such as ROSE HIP and EVENING PRIMROSE fortified with a high percentage of essential fatty acids to support collagen synthesis. Supplement face oil with anti-inflammatory and skin-regenerating essential oils such as EVERLASTING, LAVENDER, and GERANIUM. Try the GERANIUM REGENERATING SERUM on page 83. Mix 2 drops of a face oil or serum with your moisturizer for an extra-nourishing boost for your skin.

Look for a rich moisturizer containing skin-hydrating ingredients such as HYALURONIC ACID, OAT BETA GLUCAN (derived from oatmeal), and SEA ALGAE EXTRACT as well as antioxidants such as BLACK CURRANT EXTRACT, GREEN TEA EXTRACT, or vitamins A, C, and E. Apply a thin layer of a hydrating mask to your face and leave on overnight to give your skin a moisture surge. Rinse off with tepid water in the morning. Always apply sunblock to skin before going outdoors.

SKIN FITNESS

A proper diet is key for healthy mature skin. Add as many anti-oxidant foods to your diet as possible and load up on colorful fruits and vegetables rich in beta-carotene. Also, focus on foods rich in omega-3 fatty acids such as CANOLA and FLAXSEED OILS, SOY, SALMON, and other oily fish. If you enjoy spicy foods, try using TURMERIC, which has been shown to have anti-inflammatory benefits and is also a good antioxidant. Do the FOURTEEN-DAY DETOX PLAN on page 110 in the spring and fall to cleanse and renew the body. Do a follow-up WEEKEND DETOX (see page 111) as needed.

HERBAL REMEDY CHEST

HERBAL REMEDIES: Take skin-clarifying herbs such as RED CLOVER, BURDOCK, YELLOW DOCK, STINGING NETTLE, MILK THISTLE, and DANDELION, which cleanse the blood and help the liver remove toxins more efficiently. All of these herbs can be ingested as herbal extracts and added to hot water, juice, or tea or taken in capsule form.

Drink 5 cups of GREEN TEA daily.

FLOWER ESSENCES: Take appropriate FLOWER ESSENCE (see page 140) daily.

SKINCEUTICALS

Take a multivitamin daily.

Take 500 milligrams of BORAGE SEED or EVENING PRIMROSE OIL, rich in gamma linoleic acid (GLA), to help counteract oxidative stress to the skin.

SPECIAL RX

Older skin needs constant nourish-ment. Always carry a hydrolat and a small container of a replenishment cream to recharge the skin through-out the day.

Buy a humidifier for your bedroom to let your skin recharge with eight hours of moisture every night. Be sure to clean the filter regularly and add a calming essential oil to the water to help you relax.

Face oils penetrate the skin deeper than most creams do and for older skin these are a must. Select a face oil or serum fortified with essential fatty acids to plump up your skin, and do the facial massage featured on page 84 once a week.

Surround yourself with people who support a positive outlook. Find new ways to stimulate your mind and boost your creative energies, by traveling, reading, or going back to school.

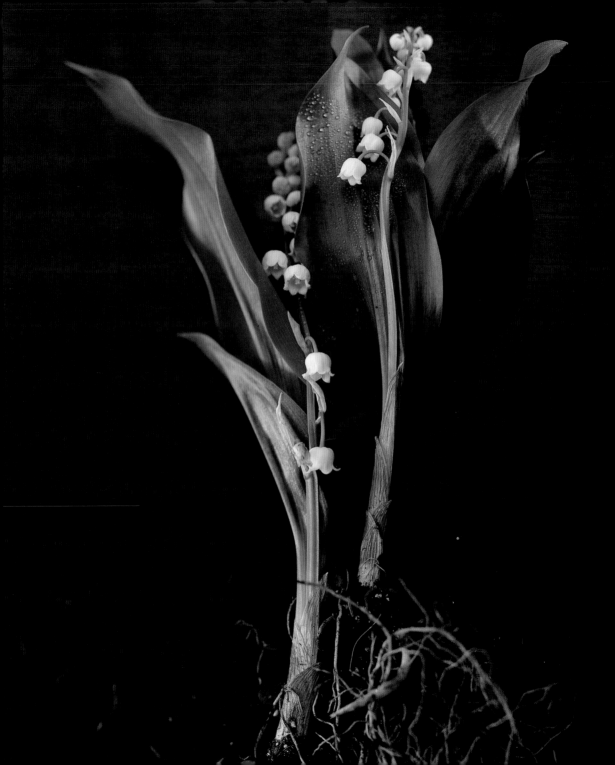

pure ingredients, pure results

SKIN-CARE RECIPES

2

It isn't easy to try to limit the amount of chemicals you put into your body. You try to eat healthy, choosing organic foods and buying filtered water. But did you know that your skin is still exposed to many other chemicals every day? Certainly many man-made products have proven invaluable in human society. But some of these innovations are simply harmful to humans, and nowhere is this more apparent than when we use harsh synthetic ingredients on our skin.

There are many natural ingredients that can be used in skin-care products instead of harsh, inert chemical ingredients. Nature offers complex and powerful ingredients whose benefits cannot be replicated in a laboratory.

A founding principle of natural medicine is that "the whole is greater than the sum of its parts." Plant extracts possess balancing secondary ingredients that help to modulate the active ingredient of the plant. Plants also contain vital energetic properties that lose their effectiveness when the ingredients are isolated. In order to receive the beneficial effects of an herb, one must take it in its entirety. And natural substances contain compounds identical to those found in the human body and therefore are recognized more easily by the body, producing enhanced results.

SAVAGE BEAUTY

With the advantages of natural products, why are harmful synthetics so prevalent? While the cosmetics industry is regulated to some degree, governmental supervision is not nearly as strict as it is for foods and drugs. Plus, synthetic ingredients are a fraction of the price of their natural counterparts, making them attractive to manufacturers. Don't be fooled by practices such as "greenwashing"—adding a few natural ingredients to a chemical-filled product—which do not give that product the benefits bestowed by nature.

INGREDIENTS TO AVOID

We can no longer view the skin as an impermeable shield. As nicotine patches have demonstrated, the skin is a permeable barrier subject to the toxicity of the ingredients we place upon it. Armed with a little knowledge, savvy consumers can steer clear of harmful or irritating products. Below are some ingredients to avoid:

DIETHANOLAMINE (DEA) **MOMOETHANOLAMINE (MEA)** **TRIETHANOLAMINE (MEA)**	Often listed on labels as Cocamide DEA, these chemicals are commonly used in cleansers, shampoos, and body washes as an emulsifier and foaming agent. According to a recent study, these chemicals affect hormone function and can have other harmful side effects.
FD&C COLOR PIGMENTS	Often made from coal tar, these artificial colorings can cause skin sensitivity and may be carcinogenic.
FRAGRANCE	Can be very sensitizing to the skin. Many of the synthetic compounds in fragrance are dangerous and can cause headaches, dizziness, or nausea.
IMIDAZOLIDINYL UREA & DMDM HYDANTOIN	These preservatives are known to cause contact dermatitis according to the American Academy of Dermatology. These preservatives also release formaldehyde, a chemical that can cause skin irritations as well as migraines, allergies, and asthma.
PETROCHEMICALS	Any petroleum-derived compounds, usually identified on labels by the prefixes or suffixes propyl-, methyl-, eth-, or -ene. Two petrochemical ingredients commonly found in skin-care products are the following: **ISOPROPYL ALCOHOL:** A petroleum-derived solvent found in hair rinses, hand lotions, and shaving products. **MINERAL OIL:** A petroleum-derived oil, sometimes marketed as baby oil, that is sensitizing to the skin and can inhibit the skin's ability to breathe.
PARABEN PRESERVATIVES	These preservatives were developed in the 1930s to stabilize creams and are now used in nearly all skin-care products. Recently researchers have found that there may be a connection between paraben preservatives and both breast cancer and male reproductive problems.
POLYETHYLENE GLYCOL (PEG)	Used to break down oil or help thicken products, this ethoxylated wetting agent for detergents, foaming agents, emulsifiers, and solvents is sometimes contaminated with 1,4-dioxane, a potential carcinogen that can penetrate the skin.
PROPYLENE GLYCOL (PG)	An alcohol that can be manufactured synthetically, usually from petroleum, or naturally, from corn. Synthetically derived, it is used as a surfactant or wetting agent. An active ingredient in industrial antifreeze, propylene glycol may cause kidney and liver abnormalities and damage cell membranes, resulting in rashes, dry skin, and surface damage to the skin.
SODIUM LAURYL SULFATE (SLS) AND SODIUM LAURETH SULFATE	These chemicals are used as surfactants to remove dirt from the skin and hair. SLS is very irritating to skin and can be toxic to eyes.

ingredients to avoid

HOW TO READ A SYNTHETIC VERSUS A NATURAL COSMETICS LABEL

Below are ingredients typically found in both a moisturizer made by a leading synthetic brand that promotes its "natural" ingredients and one made by a truly natural brand.

synthetic brand

WATER	
SQUALANE	an oil obtained through hydronation of shark's liver or plant sources
ADIPIC ACID/DIETHYLENE GLYCOL/GLYCERIN CROSSPOLYMER	a conditioner, fixative, and polymer
	an emulsifier produced synthetically from propylene alcohol
GLYCERYL STEARATE	a moisturizing agent derived from palm kernels
PEG 100 STEARATE (POLYETHYLENE GLYCOL)	a binder and emulsifier used to increase spreadability
TOCOPHERYL ACETATE	an antioxidant derived from vitamin E, often synthetically derived
RETINYL PALMITATE	a skin conditioner derived from vitamin A
AVOCADO OIL	emollient oil derived from avocado flesh, extracted with chemical solvents, decolorized, and deodorized
APRICOT KERNEL OIL	a lightweight oil derived from apricot seed, extracted with chemical solvents, decolorized, and deodorized
SWEET ALMOND OIL	a medium-weight oil, extracted with chemical solvents, decolorized, and deodorized
BEESWAX	an emulsifier, often synthetic, decolorized, and deodorized
SORBITAN OLEATE	an emulsifier derived from sugar that acts as a dispersant
STEARIC ACID	an emulsifier and thickening agent typically derived from tallow or other animal fats
MYRISTYL ALCOHOL	a mildly comedogenic and irritating emollient usually derived from coconut oil
CARBOMER	a petroleum-derived thickening and stabilizing agent that is a potential allergen
TRIETHANOLAMINE	a petroleum-derived emulsifier, possibly carcinogenic
DIAZOLIDINYL UREA	a formaldehyde-forming preservative
DISODIUM EDTA (ETHYLENE DIAMINE TETRA ACETIC ACID)	a synthetic chemical used as an antioxidant and preservative
METHYLPARABEN & PABAPARABEN	widely used preservative, possibly carcinogenic

DEIONIZED WATER	
SEA ALGAE EXTRACT	a moisturizer naturally derived from Hawaiian sea plants
APRICOT KERNEL OIL	an expeller-expressed oil that is rich in gamma linoleic acid (GLA), minerals, and vitamins; certified organic
ASCORBIC ACID POLYPEPTIDE	protein-complexed vitamin C from rose hips
OAT BETA GLUCAN	a super-moisturizer similar in efficacy to hyaluronic acid, as it helps cells retain of moisture within the skin; also provides excellent anti-inflammatory properties
SQUALANE	a lightweight oil derived from olives, wheat germ, or rice bran; also found in human sebum; certified organic
SAFFLOWER OIL	a cold-pressed oil rich in essential fatty acids
EXTRACTS OF NETTLE	an herbal infusion used for its anti-inflammatory, healing properties; certified organic
WHEAT GERM OIL	an emollient oil rich in vitamin E
ORGANIC BULGARIAN ROSE WATER	obtained during steam distillation of organic hand-picked roses and used for its soothing properties
LECITHIN	a plant phospholipid derived from soybeans, with skin-protection qualities, and used as an emulsifier and surfactant
GREEN TEA EXTRACT	counteracts irritation caused by acidic products on the skin
SUPEROXIDE DISMUTASE (SOD)	a natural liposome that allows phospholipids and vitamins to deeply penetrate lower layers of the skin
TOCOPERYL ACETATE	vitamin E, derived from wheat germ
RETINYL PALMITATE	vitamin A, which normalizes the skin's barrier properties
ASCORBIC PALMITATE	vitamin C, an active free-radical scavenger
SODIUM HYDROXYMETHYLGLYCINATE	a natural preservative derived from glycine
ALOE VERA GEL	an effective healing agent for burns; derived from the thin-walled mucilaginous cells of the plant
CALOPHYLLUM INOPHYLLUM	a cold-pressed, pale-green vegetable oil traditionally used to treat skin burns and rashes because of its ability to strengthen connective tissues
PURE ESSENTIAL OILS OF ROSE (ROSE OTTO), BLOOD ORANGE, LINDEN BLOSSOM	genuine essential oils
POTASSIUM SORBATE	a food-grade yeast and mold inhibitor
XANTHAN GUM	also known as corn sugar gum, a polysaccharide used in cosmetics as a thickener, emulsifier, and stabilizer

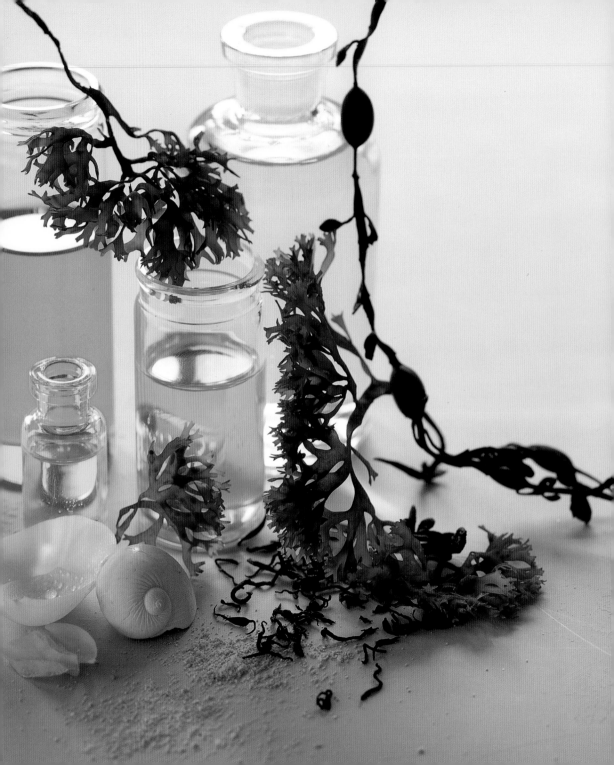

Now that you know the ingredients to avoid, you're on your way to better skin. The first step is to go to your bathroom and take a look at the labels on your current cosmetics and skin-care products. Throw away any that could be toxic. Check the expiration dates and also discard any that are more than a year old. The next step is to restock your beauty supplies with healthful products in order to get the full benefits of holistic skin care.

PURE INGREDIENTS

Nature possesses complex and powerful ingredients whose benefits cannot be replicated in a laboratory. Here is an overview of those prized natural substances that can truly benefit the skin, with no dangerous side effects. These are the building blocks for the skin-care recipes throughout the book.

ESSENTIAL OILS

Essential oils, used in aromatherapy, are derived from flowers, leaves, seeds, roots, and resins of aromatic plants to promote health and well-being. Essential oils are highly concentrated substances, often referred to as "the life force of the plant," containing chemical compounds with many antiseptic, antibiotic, analgesic, anti-inflammatory, and antiviral properties.

Holistic skin care uses clinical-grade essential oils, genuine essential oils that are not compromised by extraction with harsh solvents or through adulteration in the laboratory. Over 95 percent of the essential oils produced worldwide today are made for the perfume, food, and taste industries. These synthetic oils have no therapeutic value to the skin and actually cause skin irritation.

Essential oil molecules enter our bodies in two main ways: by inhalation or through the skin. Smelling calming scents like lavender or clary sage effects both the limbic system of the brain, the seat of emotions and memory, and also the skin, since stress has a big influence on the health of your epidermis. Because of their unique, small molecular structure and due to the fact that they are lipid (fat) soluble, essential oils can also penetrate the skin, entering the blood via the capillary network and circulating throughout the body, where they have a systemic effect.

NAME & ORIGIN	PROPERTIES & USES
BAY LAUREL *(Laurus nobilis)*	This oil stimulates and has a cleansing effect on the lymphatic system.
GERMAN CHAMOMILE *(Matricaria recutita)*	A potent anti-inflammatory oil due to high bisabolol content, this oil is excellent for burns or skin inflammations.
EVERLASTING *(Helichrysum italicum)*	A high percentage of sesquiterpenes makes this a strong anti-inflammatory oil, excellent for dry, irritated skin or broken capillaries.
GERANIUM *(Pelargonium odorantissimum)*	This oil possesses a combination of terpene alcohols and esters to give it antiseptic and balancing properties; it also produces a strong relaxing effect on the central nervous system.
JUNIPER *(Juniperus communis)*	This stimulating oil has antiseptic qualities, making it useful in skin care.
LAVENDER *(Lavandula vera or Lavandula angustifolia)*	Lavender comes in many forms and is excellent for toning the skin and promoting relaxation.
LEMON VERBENA *(Lippia citriodora)*	This member of the citrus family has a high citral content, which makes it one of the most calming and relaxing aromatherapeutic oils.
NEROLI *(Citrus aurantium)*	High linolol, linalyl acetate, and geraniol content give this oil its balancing and soothing properties, especially useful in regulating sebum production.
ROSE *(Rose otto damascena)*	Citronellol and geraniol give this oil its soothing and balancing properties. Excellent for calming down irritated skin as well as relaxing the central nervous system.
ROSEMARY *(Rosmarinus officinalis or Rosmarinus verbanone)*	The verbanone type is ideal for skin care due to its skin cell regenerating properties.
TEA TREE *(Melaleuca alternifolia)*	Well known for its antiseptic and antiviral properties due to high terpene alcohol content, this oil is beneficial for oily and acne-prone skin.
THYME *(Thymus vulgaris)* **LINALOOL TYPE**	This type of thyme oil has strong antiseptic qualities but is gentle enough to be used on the skin to treat impurities.

SKIN PERSONALITY	COMMENTS
B HR SR ER M	
SR ER M	Bright blue color is the hallmark of this oil.
SR ER M	
B HR SR ER M	This oil is often adulterated so be sure to purchase from a reputable supplier.
HR	
B HR SR ER M	Varieties grown in high alpine regions of France or Croatia have a high linolol content, making them very antiseptic and especially useful on oily or acne-prone skin and on burns. The lowland varieties, found in the Grasse region of France, contain a high ester content, making it a powerful relaxing oil, useful for stress-related conditions.
B HR SR ER M	This oil is often adulterated so be sure to purchase from a reputable supplier.
B HR SR ER M	This oil is produced from the small, white flowers of the bitter-orange tree.
B HR SR ER M	An expensive oil to distill due to the large number of rose petals needed to yield a significant amount of oil.
B HR SR ER M	Genuine rosemary oil is usually cultivated in France or Spain and has a high camphor content, making it a superlative relaxing oil for use in massage.
HR	Tea Tree is also useful for the treatment of cold sores, herpes, and nail fungus.
HR	

hydrolats

Hydrolats, also called floral waters, are a by-product of the steam distillation process used to extract essential oils. When plant material such as lavender is exposed to steam, volatile therapeutic components are released into the water. The essential oil is then drawn off, leaving the hydrosol, which contains molecules of essential oils and constituents from the herb or flower. Like homeopathic medicines, these waters possess a vibrational energy that can be used to help balance and fortify the skin. Below are some of the commonly available hydrolats:

ROSE
  (Rosa damascena)
  calms; soothes redness

NEROLI
  (Citrus aurantium)
  balances; assists in sebum
  regulation

LAVENDER
  (Lavandula vera)
  antiseptic; good for oiliness,
  blemishes

GERMAN CHAMOMILE
  (Matricaria recutita)
  anti-inflammatory;
  calms irritated skin

VEGETAL OILS

Carrier oils are an important element in therapeutic aromatherapy and skin care. Due to their high concentration, essential oils need to be diluted in a carrier or base oil before they are applied to the skin. But a carrier oil does much more than just act as a vehicle to deliver essential oils to the skin—it can make all the difference between a low- and high-quality skin-care product.

Certainly a mineral oil, petrolatum, or paraffin wax can do the job satisfactorily—and very inexpensively. However, these by-products of petrochemical industry processing are inert carriers that do not let the skin breathe. In contrast, vegetal oils, made from nuts and seeds such as almonds, hazelnuts, and sunflowers offer a wide spectrum of nutritional benefits to the skin, and they help build the membranes that support the cell structure.

Vegetal oils also contain many organic compounds that enhance skin functioning and heal the body, such as essential fatty acids (especially gamma linoleic acid, or GLA, essential for collagen production), phospholipids (in particular, lecithin, which acts as an emulsifier), phytosterols (plant hormones), and antioxidant carotenes and vitamins.

These properties are the reason that vegetal oils have long been used around the world for their ability to heal the body. In Madagascar, Hawaii, and Tahiti, the vegetal oil calophyllum inophyllum has been used to treat skin conditions such as burns and rashes because of its ability to strengthen connective tissues. In Central Africa, shea butter, a natural fat obtained from the nuts of the karate tree, is prized for its skin-softening effects and is also known to increase epidermal thickness due to moisture-retaining properties. It is also a common remedy used for treating stretch marks.

To make high-quality skin-care products using vegetal oils, you'll need to make sure the oils have been processed correctly. The best vegetal oils are produced by heating them gently at low temperatures so that excessive heat does not kill the valuable elements in the oil. They are processed without chemical extraction, and without solvents like hexane.

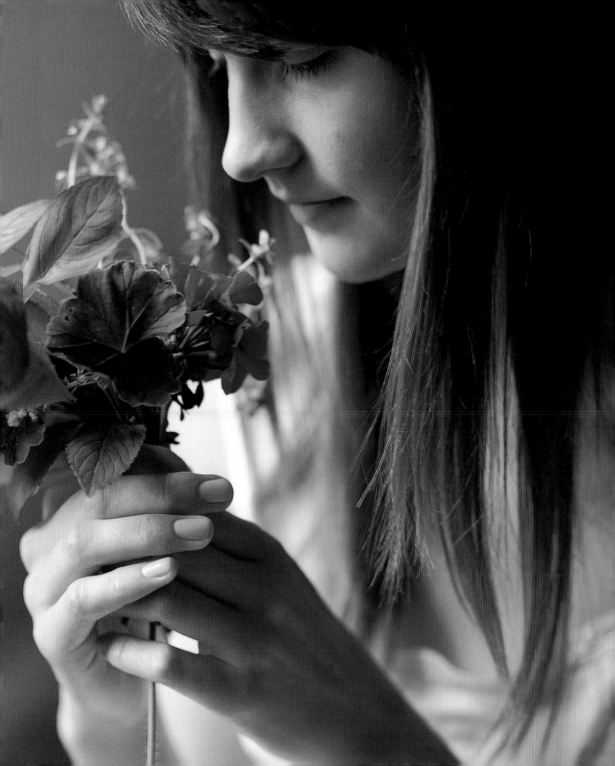

NAME	PROPERTIES & USES
SWEET ALMOND OIL	High fatty acid content makes it good for creams. Oil does not disperse well and is too heavy to be used alone for massage.
APRICOT KERNEL OIL	High fatty acid content helps devitalized skin. Light texture good for face serums, especially for oily skin.
ARNICA OIL	Anti-inflammatory oil, excellent for bruises, sprains, or sore muscles.
AVOCADO OIL	Flesh of fruit yields emollient, full-bodied oil, good for dry, dull skin.
BLACK CURRANT SEED OIL	High GLA content supports collagen synthesis and improves skin elasticity.
BORAGE SEED OIL	High GLA content ideal for skin conditions such as eczema as well as for stretch marks and prematurely aged skin.
CALENDULA OIL	Wound-healing properties make this oil good for inflamed skin.
EVENING PRIMROSE OIL	High GLA content makes this oil indispensable in skin care especially for mature or dry, irritated skin and conditions such as eczema and psoriasis.
HAZELNUT OIL	Fine-textured oil is highly penetrative; good for face serums, especially on oily skin.
JOJOBA OIL	Similarity to human sebum makes this oil excellent in face oils.
MACADAMIA OIL	Light, penetrating oil ideal for face serums. Palmitoleic acid helps delay skin aging due to essential fatty acid content.
ROSE HIP SEED OIL	This is a superb cell-regenerative and tissue-healing oil due to high EFA content. Excellent for scar healing and for treating prematurely aged skin.
SUNFLOWER OIL	This oil is most commonly used as the base for macerated oils. It has a light texture, similar to human sebum.
WHEAT GERM OIL	Natural antioxidant often used to stabilize serum and massage blends.

SKIN PERSONALITY

COMMENTS

Skin Personality	Comments
B, SR, ER, M	For body massage, dilute with lighter-weight base oil such as safflower or sunflower.
HR	Can be used undiluted.
B, HR, SR, ER, M	Use as an addition to a base oil, such as almond, safflower, or sunflower (10 percent of the whole).
B, SR, ER, M	Use as an addition to a base oil, such as almond, safflower, or sunflower (10 percent of the whole).
M	Use as an addition to a base oil, such as almond, safflower, or sunflower (10 percent of the whole).
SR, ER, M	Use as an addition to a base oil, such as almond, safflower, or sunflower (10 percent of the whole).
SR, ER, M	Use as an addition to a base oil, such as almond, safflower, or sunflower (10 percent of the whole).
SR, ER, M	Use as an addition to a base oil, such as almond, safflower, or sunflower (10 percent of the whole).
B, HR, SR, ER, M	Can be used undiluted.
B, HR, SR, ER, M	Can be used undiluted but is usually used as an addition to a base oil such as almond, safflower, or sunflower (30 percent of the whole).
M	Can be used undiluted.
SR, ER, M	Use as an addition to a base oil such as almond, safflower, or sunflower (20 percent of the whole).
B, HR, SR, ER, M	Can be used undiluted. Suitable base oil for body massage.
B, HR, SR, ER, M	Use as an addition to a base oil such as almond, safflower, or sunflower (10 percent of the whole).

KEY

B BALANCED   HR HORMONE REACTIVE   SR STRESS REACTIVE   ER ENVIRONMENT REACTIVE   M MATURE

HERBAL EXTRACTS

Extracts can be derived from a variety of plants, herbs, flowers, and sea plants and are usually made by infusing them in an alcohol or glycerin base. These extracts are very concentrated and can have a variety of therapeutic properties. Following are some of the more common herbal extracts:

herbal extracts

NAME	PROPERTIES & USES
ALOE VERA	Derived from the thin-walled mucilaginous cells of the plant, aloe vera gel is an effective healing agent for burns, as well as a superior humectant due to its ability to attract moisture to the skin.
CONEFLOWER (ECHINACEA) EXTRACT	This extract is very effective when used topically as a skin tonic to dilate peripheral blood vessels and reduce inflammation.
GREEN TEA EXTRACT	Known as an internal remedy for its antioxidant properties, it is also useful as an external remedy, counteracting irritation caused by acidic products.
MEADOWSWEET EXTRACT	Rich in vitamin C, this herb contains salicylic acid and citric acid.
NETTLE EXTRACT	An herbal infusion useful for its anti-inflammatory properties, especially in healing rashes and burns.
OAT BETA GLUCAN	A super-moisturizer that forms a thin invisible film to help retention of moisture within the skin. It also provides excellent anti-inflammatory properties.
RED GRAPE SEED EXTRACT	A source of proanthocyanidins and flavonoids, which protect capillary walls and inhibit the enzymes that break down collagen and elastin. It also acts as an anti-inflammatory agent and as a major free-radical scavenger.
RED WINE EXTRACT	Rich in resveratrol, an antioxidant and free-radical scavenger that stimulates cellular proliferation and collagen synthesis.
SEA ALGAE EXTRACT	This excellent moisturizer leaves the skin feeling smoother and silkier but may cause a significant thickening of the epidermis.
SHEA BUTTER	Has a softening effect on the skin and counteracts dehydration of the skin.

SKIN PERSONALITY	COMMENTS

SKIN PERSONALITY

B	HR	SR	ER	M

Studies indicate that aloe vera gel, when applied, increases the production of cells in the dermis layer of the skin, which in turn produces collagen to keep skin firm and supple.

SR	ER	M

Research indicates that echinacea is effective in healing cuts, burns, eczema, and psoriasis due to its blood-cleansing abilities.

B	HR	SR	ER	M

B	HR	SR	ER	M

SR	ER

B	HR	SR	ER	M

In laboratory experiments, oat beta glucan appears to stimulate the immune system, right down to the cell level. It protects against UVA induced oxidative stress, reduces transepidermal water loss, and restores skin function.

B	HR	SR	ER	M

M

B	HR	SR	ER	M

Make sure the seaweed extract you use does not contain iodine, a potential skin irritant.

B	SR	ER	M

A natural fat obtained from the nuts of the karate tree in Central Africa.

KEY

B BALANCED	HR HORMONE REACTIVE	SR STRESS REACTIVE	ER ENVIRONMENT REACTIVE	M MATURE

NATURAL FRUIT ACIDS AND ENZYMES

Fruit acids such as alpha hydroxy acids (AHAs), glycolic acids, and enzymes are helpful in the exfoliation of dead skin cells, thereby promoting the proliferation of new skin cells. Both fruit acids and enzymes are naturally occurring substances found in many common fruits and other foods such as pumpkins, cherries, pomegranates, pineapples, papayas, and grapes; lactic acid, similar to fruit acid, comes from sour milk. Glycolic acid is naturally derived from sugarcane.

AHAs, enzymes, and glycolic acids work by breaking down the protein bonds making up the superficial layers of the skin. This loosening of the outer layer of skin leads to a gentle exfoliation of the dead skin cells. As these skin cells are sloughed off, the process of making new skin cells is accelerated, giving the skin a fresher, healthier appearance. However, care must be taken not to overuse these acids and enzymes, so that the integrity of the skin is maintained. Because this exfoliation process thins the outer layer of the skin, always apply sunscreen before you go outdoors.

NATURAL PRESERVATIVES

There are alternatives to the irritating and potentially toxic preservatives used in mass-produced skin-care products. Grapefruit seed extract, essential oils, and vitamin E, as well as food-grade preservatives such as potassium sorbate, citric acid, and cinnamon-oil and glycerin derivatives, have all proven to be effective preservatives, to varying degrees. You may not even need a preservative at all, as when you make products such as bath and body oils, bath salts, and salves.

SKIN FOOD: MAKING YOUR OWN SKIN CARE PREPARATIONS

This next section focuses on the building blocks of homemade skin-care products, first identifying the individual components and then providing you with recipes for making your own custom-designed skin-care products right in your own kitchen.

Making your own cosmetics at home can be both easy and fun and has the added benefit of allowing you to know exactly what you are using on your skin. You will discover that these recipes do not have to be complicated in order to be effective. All you will need is some basic equipment and a handful of ingredients easily found at your local hardware, grocery, and health food store (or see the resources section at the back of this book).

RAW MATERIALS

In order for your skin-care preparations to be effective, they need to be made using high-quality ingredients. If something is selling cheaply, there is usually a reason. For example, vanilla fragrance costs $6 a pound, but genuine, certified-organic vanilla costs approximately $1,400 a pound (don't worry—you will only need a few drops!). High-quality natural ingredients will always cost more because the plant from which they came was cultivated without the use of pesticides or handpicked in the wild, both of which processes are very labor intensive. In addition, these very same plants are subject to droughts, weather shifts, and insects, making consistent, large yields difficult to achieve. The good news is that a plant or herb that has withstood these conditions is always hardier and possesses more therapeutic value, and this is exactly what nature intended: survival of the fittest. Check the resources section in the back of the book for a list of reputable suppliers of essential oils, herbal oils, and natural raw materials that you can trust to deliver the best ingredients.

The following pages provide you with the basic procedures you'll want to use to create your own skin-care and body-care products.

BASIC EQUIPMENT

Atomizer sprayer

Blender or food processor

Colored glass bottles
in assorted sizes

Double boiler
or saucepan with Pyrex
or metal bowl

Food scale

French coffee press

Glass or ceramic jars
in assorted sizes

Grater

Hand whisk

Measuring cup

Mixing bowls (large and small)

Muslin (cheesecloth)

Mortar and pestle

Strainer

Tea kettle

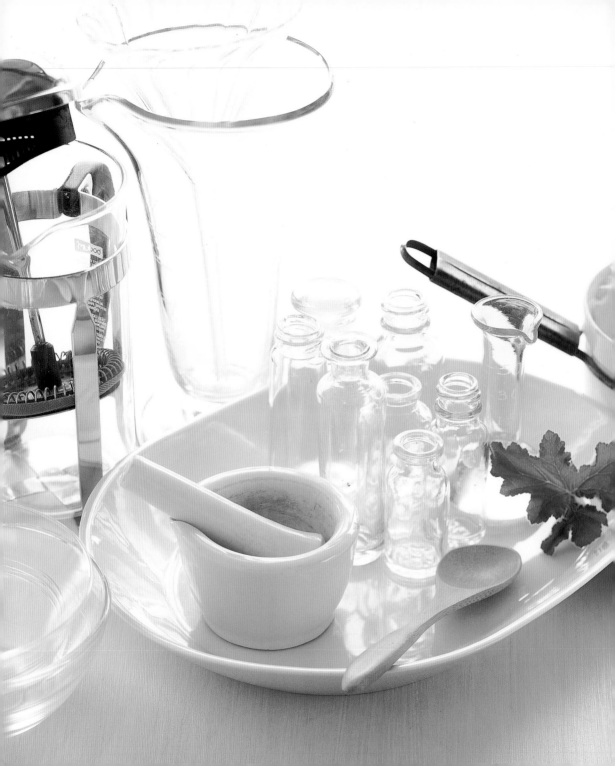

ESSENTIAL OILS

As a general rule, essential oils need to be diluted before you apply them to the skin. The two exceptions to this rule are lavender and tea tree oils, which are gentle enough to be applied neat to the skin.

The way in which essential oils are blended, and the carrier oils or base creams selected, will very much depend on the condition you are treating. As a general rule of thumb when making blends, you will want to use no more than 3 percent essential oils in the total carrier oil. Products intended for the face will have a lower percentage of essential oil than those intended for the body.

Blending is both an art and a science that requires practice while you build up familiarity not only with the therapeutic properties of essential oils but also with their fragrances. A good way to learn how to do this is to follow the blending basics outlined on page 64. These guidelines can help you decide which essential and carrier oils to use and keep track of the amounts of each oil you have selected, for future reference. It may take several tries to get the exact formula that you want. This is the fun part of natural-skin-care alchemy.

The basic rule for blending is to combine no more than a total of four or five essential oils in a blend. An ideal amount is usually three or four oils; with more than four the blend begins to get crowded and loses its effectiveness. Select your essential oils in order of therapeutic value. The first will make up the largest percentage of the blend. The second will make up the next largest portion, and so on.

Next, you'll choose a carrier oil. You can select one oil or choose to fortify your blend with a specialty oil such as evening primrose or arnica oil to boost the therapeutic value of your blend (the vegetal oil chart on pages 56-57 can help you decide how much of the oil to use).

Once you have combined your essential and carrier oils together and have completed the blend, let the mixture stand for at least an hour (or overnight) to let the oils "cook" or amalgamate. You will find that giving the mixture some additional time before using it will allow the oils to open up creating a more powerful synergistic effect as well as a smoother aromatic bouquet.

Essential oils are light sensitive and so should be stored in dark colored bottles. Plastics should never be used because certain oils are very aggressive and can corrode plastic. Cobalt and amber glass bottles can easily be found at a hardware store or from the specialty aromatherapy suppliers listed in the back of this book.

AROMATHERAPY BLENDING BASICS

Follow these guidelines each time you create a blend. When you begin creating your own blends, it is easy to use too much of one oil or not enough of another. This template helps you to break down that process so you can achieve the optimum results.

TREATMENT GOAL:

On a sheet of paper, list what your treatment objectives are — nourish dry skin, clear up blemishes, reduce scarring, and so on. For example, to treat stress-induced insomnia the treatment goal might be: BLEND A CALMING NIGHTTIME BATH OIL.

ESSENTIAL OILS:

List the essential oils selected and why. You can use one essential oil or create a blend using no more than five oils. For example, to create the bath oil mentioned above some possible treatment oils might be:

LAVENDER, MANDARIN, SANDALWOOD, and ROSE.

CARRIER OILS OR LOTION:

List the carrier oil(s) or lotion chosen and why. List the percentage or proportion of each oil used in the blend. For example, for a bath oil you might want a blend of lightweight oils that will not feel heavy on the skin or leave a tub residue, such as:

WALNUT ($\frac{1}{3}$), ALMOND ($\frac{1}{3}$), and SUNFLOWER ($\frac{1}{3}$).

BLENDING NOTES:

Fill the bottle halfway with the blend of carrier oils. Figure out the total number of drops of essential oils (4-ounce bottle = total 50 drops, 2-ounce bottle = total 25 drops, 1-ounce bottle = 12 drops). Then list here each of the essential oils as follows:

LAVENDER: 18 ~~卌 卌 卌~~ |||
MANDARIN: 14 ~~卌 卌~~ ||||
SANDALWOOD: 12 ~~卌 卌~~ ||
ROSE: 6 ~~卌~~ |
TOTAL: 50 drops
4-ounce bottle

BLENDING ESSENTIAL OILS

To figure out how many drops of each essential oil to use, begin with your "lead" oil (the one you feel has the greatest therapeutic power to treat the condition) and add what you think is the best number of drops to achieve your goal. Place that number of hatch marks next to the name of that oil. Repeat with the remaining oils, close the bottle and agitate. Smell the oil. If you feel that the fragrance is not quite right, adjust by adding more of a particular oil and document the addition by making the appropriate number of hatch marks next to that oil. When the blend seems right, top off the bottle with carrier oil. Agitate a second time.

Use the following chart as your reference guide when blending essential oils:

NAME	BLENDING INSTRUCTIONS
FACE SERUM	Fill a 2-ounce bottle halfway with a lightweight carrier oil such as apricot kernel, hazelnut, or jojoba oil. Add 20 drops total of essential oils. Close the bottle and roll it between your hands to disperse the oils. Top off with carrier oil. Agitate a second time.
MASSAGE OIL	Fill a 4-ounce bottle halfway with a blend of medium-weight oils that provide good slippage, such as almond, safflower, sunflower, and walnut oil. Add 40 to 50 drops total of essential oils. Close bottle and roll it between hands to disperse the oils. Top off with carrier oil. Agitate a second time.
BATH OIL	Follow the instructions for massage oil, above.
BODY LOTION	Fill a 4-ounce bottle one-third full of an unscented lotion or cream made of natural base materials. Add 25 drops total of essential oils, close the bottle, and shake well. Uncap and add another third of lotion or cream. Add 25 more drops of essential oils, replace lid and shake well. Top off with remaining third of lotion or cream. Agitate a final time.

blending essential oils

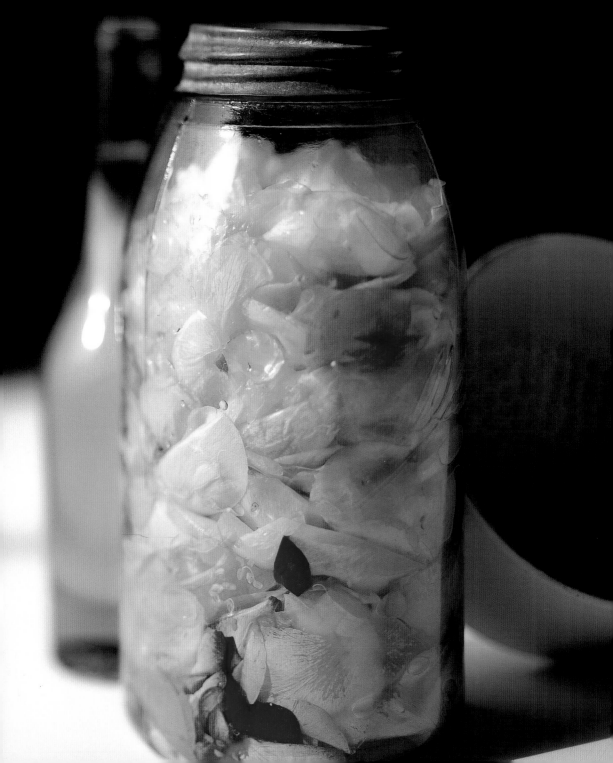

HERBAL OILS

Adding herbs to a base, or carrier, oil can enhance the therapeutic properties of that oil. The flowers or herbs are lightly bruised and steeped in a carrier oil, most commonly safflower or sunflower oil, each of which absorbs easily into the skin. Solar-infused herbal oils use the heat of the sun to gently warm the oil; flowering plants such as arnica, calendula, and St. John's wort are ideal for use in solar-infused herbal oils. Simmering is the preferred extraction method for the leaves of herbs such as rosemary and comfrey, since more intense heat is required to pull the active materials from the plant. These oils will keep for up to twelve months and can be added to carrier oils or lotions.

SOLAR HERBAL OILS

Solar-infused herbal oils are fun to make in the summer, when there is an abundance of fresh plant material, and the long, hot days of summer can assist in the production of the oil. In addition to the herbs mentioned above, any number of flowering plants can be used, such as CALENDULA, MEADOW-SWEET, LAVENDER, and ROSE.

CALENDULA INFUSED OIL

MAKES 1 QUART

fresh calendula (*Calendula officinalis*) flower heads
to fill two jars
16 ounces safflower oil

32-ounce colored glass bottle

PREP TIME:
1 HOUR
(plus time for
solar infusion)

Harvest the calendula flowers on a sunny day and discard any soiled parts of the plant. Do not wash the flower heads, since the water would encourage mold to grow. Using your hands, gently bruise or break the flowers to extract as much active plant material as possible. Densely pack a 1-quart canning jar to the brim with calendula flower heads and cover completely with oil to the rim of the jar. Place lid tightly on the jar, label with the name of the plant and the date, and leave on a sunny windowsill or in a greenhouse for 2 to 3 weeks.

Using a cheesecloth or muslin bag, strain the mixture into a container. Now repeat the process by densely packing another 1-quart canning jar with bruised fresh calendula flower tops and fill to the brim with the once-infused oil. Cap the jar and let steep for an additional 2 to 3 weeks. Strain the mixture once again through a cheesecloth or muslin bag and store in a colored glass bottle.

Add solar-infused oil to any blend (3 to 10 percent of the total).

SIMMERED HERBAL OILS

Use this method when you're working with plant leaves, roots, or any woody material that may be more difficult to extract.

MAKES 1 QUART

ROSEMARY HERBAL OIL

PREP TIME:
2 HOURS 30 MINUTES

2 cups fresh rosemary leaves
16 ounces safflower oil

1-quart canning jar

Gently bruise or break the rosemary leaves to extract as much active plant material as possible. Put the oil and the rosemary in a double boiler or heatproof glass bowl set over a pan of simmering water. Gently heat the mixture for 2 hours and then strain through cheesecloth or muslin bag into canning jar.

Add simmered oils to any blend (3 to 10 percent of the total).

HERBAL INFUSIONS

Extracts can be made from plants using a variety of solvents to pull out the active ingredients. When water is used as a solvent, the end product is tea. Herbal infusions can be made with fresh or dried herbs and can be added to creams or balms for the herbs' therapeutic properties. Herbs that can easily be used in infusions include GREEN TEA, ROSEMARY, BORAGE, CALENDULA, CHAMOMILE, LEMON BALM, GERANIUM, and ROSE PETALS.

HERBAL INFUSION

MAKES 1 CUP

2 ounces fresh (or 1 ounce dried) herbs, bruised
1 cup distilled water

1-quart canning jar

PREP TIME:
15 MINUTES

Place the herbs in a French press. In a small pan, bring distilled water to a boil on the stove and pour over the herbs. Let the tea steep for 10 minutes. Strain and pour into canning jar.

Use this mixture to supplement creams or balms or add herbal infusions to bath water to enhance the therapeutic effect of the bath.

HERBAL DECOCTIONS

Herbal decoctions are made by **boiling** the **roots, bark, berries, seeds,** and **woodier** parts of a plant in water to extract the active ingredients. This usually requires a longer extraction time than is needed for teas due to the nature of the material. Plants that can be extracted in herbal decoctions include BURDOCK ROOT, DEVIL'S CLAW, ECHINACEA ROOT, and GINSENG.

MAKES 3 CUPS

PREP TIME:
45 MINUTES

HERBAL DECOCTION

1 ounce fresh herbs (or ½ ounce dried herbs)

4 cups distilled water

1-quart canning jar

Break up plant material by crushing it using a mortar and pestle or chopping with a knife. Place herbs and distilled water in a saucepan and allow the water to boil for about 15 minutes, until it has been reduced to approximately 3 cups. Cover and steep for an additional 10 minutes. Strain into canning jar and let cool. Decoctions will last 3 or 4 days in refrigerator.

Use this mixture to supplement creams or balms or add herbal decoctions to bath water to enhance the therapeutic effect of the bath.

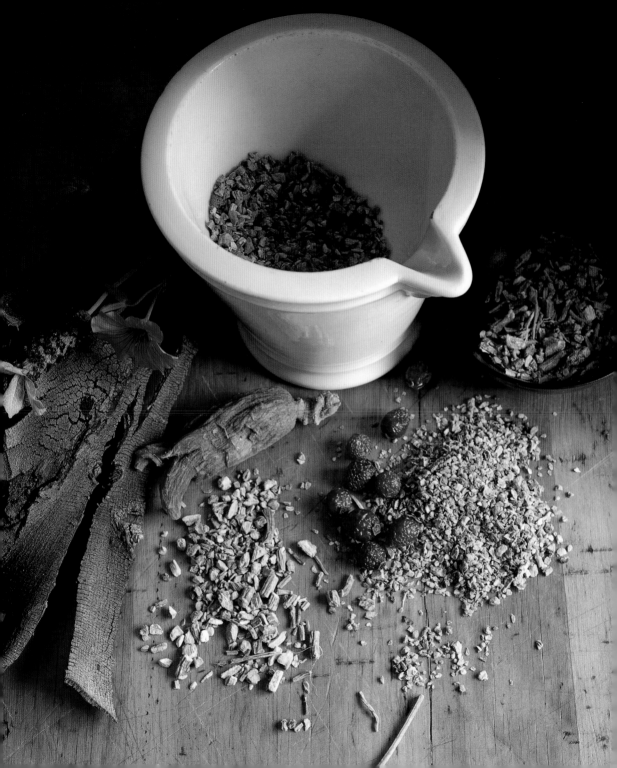

THE RECIPES

Now that you know the basics of natural skin care, you're ready to try **making some of your own all-natural skin-care products.** The essential oils and herbal derivatives described in the previous section form the building blocks for cleansers and moisturizers for the face and skin.

CLEANSERS

Cleansing is the most important step of your skin-care regimen, so you want to make sure that you are not using an aggressive surfactant that would strip the good oils from your skin. Most skin imbalances are caused by overcleansing of the skin, since we have been conditioned to believe that only harsh, foamy cleaners are effective. This creates a whole host of problems as the skin tries to correct itself. Nature provides excellent alternatives to synthetic cleansing products. Try these gentle cleansers, made with ANTISEPTIC ESSENTIAL OILS and ORGANIC BASE MATERIALS.

CLARIFYING CLEANSING OIL

SKIN PERSONALITY

B   HR   SR   ER   M

This cleansing oil contains antiseptic essential oils to eliminate blackheads. The vegetal oil base is perfect for removing oil-based makeup.

MAKES 2 OUNCES

PREP TIME:
15 MINUTES

1½ ounces apricot kernel oil
10 drops rosemary (*Rosemarinus officinalis*) essential oil
6 drops lavender (*Lavandula vera*) essential oil
4 drops cypress (*Cupressus sempervirens*) essential oil
½ ounce jojoba oil

2-ounce glass bottle

Fill bottle with apricot kernel oil. Add essential oils, close bottle, and roll between hands to disperse oils. Top off with jojoba oil. Close bottle and agitate a second time.

Rinse face with warm water. Apply a small amount of cleansing oil to pads of fingers or cotton pad and wipe over the face and throat area, gently loosening any makeup or grime. Rinse off with cool water.

CLEANSING FACIAL GOMAGE

This rich cleansing cream is suited for drier complexions or those skin personalities that need a more delicate cleansing regimen. The milk from the oats contains salicylic acid to soothe irritated skin and the baking soda will leave your skin silky and smooth.

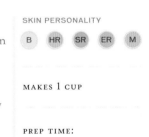

SKIN PERSONALITY

B HR SR ER M

MAKES 1 CUP

PREP TIME:
30 MINUTES

    With this recipe you also have the option of adding superfine pastry sugar to turn the formula into a scrub. As the skin gradually renews itself every month, some of the old cells may stick to the surface of the skin longer than they should. As a result, your skin may have a dull and sometimes flaky appearance, and those dead cells may clog the pores and lead to blemishes. A good exfoliation helps to push this natural regeneration process along and keep your skin soft and clear.

> ¼ cup chamomile or calendula herbal infusion
>   (see page 69)
> ¼ cup oats
> 1 teaspoon baking soda
> 1 tablespoon honey
> 2 tablespoons superfine sugar (optional)

Prepare the herbal infusion and let steep. Combine oats, baking soda, and honey together in a mixing bowl. Pour herbal infusion over oat mixture, add superfine sugar if desired, combine well, and set aside for 5 minutes.

Rinse face with warm water. Apply a small amount of cleansing gomage to pads of fingers and gently massage all over face, taking care not to overstimulate the skin by scrubbing too long. Discard leftover gomage.

CLARIFYING FACIAL SAUNA

SKIN PERSONALITY

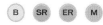

MAKES 2 CUPS

PREP TIME:
15 MINUTES

Contrary to popular belief, a facial steam bath does not open pores. Pores do not fluctuate in size, but they do fill up with dirt and debris. A good facial steam with antiseptic and stimulating essential oils and herbs helps to promote circulation and soften the skin, making the process of removing impurities much more easy.

1 ounce fresh rosemary leaves, bruised
1 ounce fresh basil leaves, bruised
1 sprig fresh thyme, bruised
4 drops lavender (*Lavandula vera*) essential oil

Combine all the herbs in a French press. Pour boiling water over herbs. Let steep for 10 minutes. Keep tea kettle filled with boiling water to add extra heat to your facial steam.

Fill the clean bathroom sink with hot tap water. Place 4 drops of lavender essential oil in water and swish with hand to disperse oil. Add herbal infusion from French press to water in sink. Cover head and shoulders with a towel and lean over the basin, making a tent to hold in the steam. Add more hot water from kettle as needed.

TONERS

Toners not only help adjust the pH level but also can help remove any traces of dirt left after cleansing. The best toners are hydrolats, since these homeopathic waters, which are a by-product of the steam distillation of essential oils, contain micronized particles of essential oils that penetrate the skin to deliver therapeutic results. In the following recipes, essential oils are added to distilled water in order to nourish and balance the skin.

GREEN TEA TONER

Green tea is well known for its antioxidant properties and aloe vera acts as a humectant to draw moisture into the skin. Use this toner after cleansing to recharge your skin and make it glow.

1 teaspoon dried peppermint leaves
4 teaspoons green tea leaves
4 ounces distilled water
2 drops lavender (*Lavandula vera*) essential oil
2 teaspoons aloe vera gel

4-ounce bottle with spray atomizer

SKIN PERSONALITY

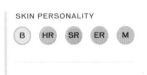
B HR SR ER M

MAKES 4 OUNCES

PREP TIME:
15 MINUTES

Combine the herbs in a French press. In a small pan, bring distilled water to a rolling boil and pour over herbs. Add lavender essential oil, let steep for 10 minutes, plunge, and let cool. Pour aloe vera gel into bottle and fill with herbal infusion. Cap with spray atomizer.

Spritz face liberally. Keep in refrigerator for added soothing benefits.

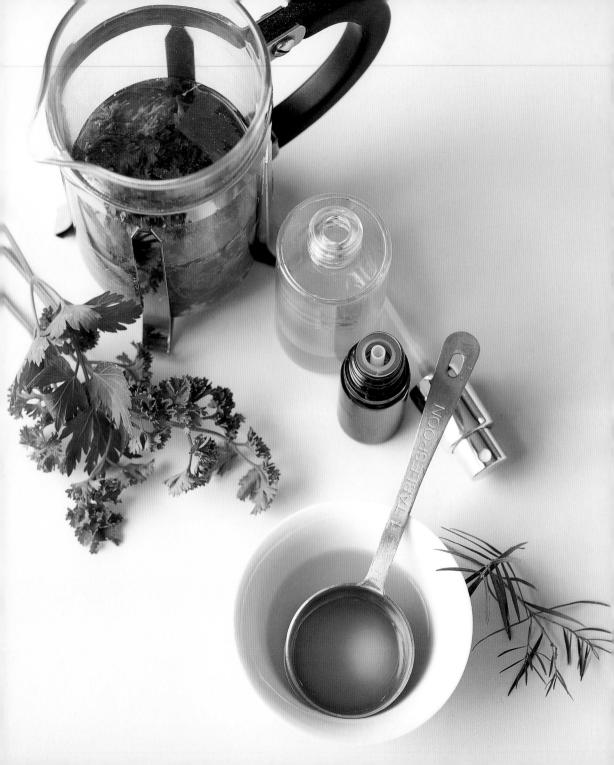

CLARIFYING PARSLEY TONER

This toner is excellent for skin that is hormone reactive or prone to breakouts and blemishes. PARSLEY is a clarifying herb and TEA TREE has strong antiseptic properties that help to clear up blemishes. APPLE CIDER VINEGAR is also an important blemish fighter because it has a high acid content and the bacteria that cause blemishes cannot thrive in an acidic environment.

SKIN PERSONALITY

HR

MAKES 4 OUNCES

PREP TIME:
20 MINUTES

1 ounce fresh parsley leaves, bruised
½ cup distilled water
1 tablespoon apple cider vinegar
4 drops tea tree oil

4-ounce bottle with spray atomizer

Place the parsley in a French press. In a small pan, bring distilled water to a rolling boil and pour over the parsley. Let steep for 10 minutes, plunge, and let cool. Pour apple cider vinegar and tea tree oil into bottle and top off with parsley infusion. Cap with spray atomizer and shake well.

Spritz face liberally. Keep in refrigerator for added soothing benefits.

PLANT MILK

SKIN PERSONALITY

SR ER

MAKES 4 OUNCES

PREP TIME:
20 MINUTES

This recipe is good for use in the wintertime when your skin is feeling raw or exposed, or any time your skin feels dry or sensitive. This plant milk is derived from OATS, a natural skin soother, and also contains CALENDULA, a traditional anti-inflammatory herb. It will leave the skin feeling soft and moisturized.

1 ounce dried calendula flowers
½ cup oats
8 ounces distilled water

4-ounce bottle with spray atomizer

Combine the calendula and oats in a French press. In a small pan bring distilled water to a rolling boil and pour water over herbs and oats. Let steep for 10 minutes, plunge, and let cool. Pour into bottle, and cap with spray atomizer.

Spritz face liberally. Keep in refrigerator for added soothing benefits.

MOISTURIZERS AND SERUMS

All moisturizers are simply an emulsion of oil and water. The purpose is twofold: to draw moisture into the skin and seal it in (this is why it is always a good idea to put on a moisturizer on right after you have cleaned your face, while the skin is still damp) and to nourish and support the outer layers of the skin by filling up the gaps between the skin cells. In this respect, natural creams outshine their synthetic counterparts because, due to their similarity to the composition of human skin, they are more easily absorbed.

You can buy all-natural base creams and lotions from a natural skin-care supplier (see Resources, page 142). I don't recommend making creams at home, as it is not possible to achieve the smooth texture of a professionally made natural cream, and because homemade creams will need to be refrigerated. Alternatively, plant serums are easy to prepare at home and deliver the results you need.

Traditionally the word *serum* meant the blood serum of an animal used as a therapeutic agent. Today, plant serums are used in holistic skin care because they contain natural amino acids that help to regulate and condition the skin and are essential in correcting skin imbal-ances and revitalizing a dull complexion. Think of plant serums as your custom-blended skin conditioners.

NEROLI TONING SERUM

SKIN PERSONALITY

(B)

MAKES 2 OUNCES

PREP TIME:
20 MINUTES

The blossoming flowers of NEROLI and YLANG-YLANG give this serum its rich, luxurious scent. The antiseptic properties of THYME and the skin-cell-regenerating power of ROSEMARY VERBENONE make this an ideal daily maintenance oil for balanced skin.

1 ounce hazelnut or apricot kernel oil
6 drops neroli (*Citrus aurantium*) essential oil
5 drops ylang-ylang (*Cananga odorata*) essential oil
6 drops rosemary verbenone (*Rosmarinus officinalis,* verbenone type) essential oil
3 drops thyme (*Thymus vulgaris,* linalool type) essential oil
1 ounce jojoba oil

2-ounce glass bottle

Fill bottle halfway with hazelnut oil. Add essential oils, close bottle, and roll bottle between palms to disperse the oils. Top off with jojoba oil, close bottle, and agitate a second time.

Cleanse and tone skin. Apply 3 or 4 drops to a cotton pad or fingertips and wipe over entire face. To plump up the skin, use serum in conjunction with facial massage (see page 84).

CARROT SEED PROTECTIVE SERUM

This serum is beneficial for **calming** and **nourishing** dry or sensitive skin. The combination of soothing VEGETAL OILS, AVOCADO, and EVENING PRIMROSE **revitalizes** dull skin with a high concentration of vitamins and essential fatty acids. The regenerating and **stimulating** properties of CARROT SEED and ROSEMARY VERBENONE essential oils help to bring the skin back to life.

1⅓ ounce hazelnut or apricot kernel oil
5 drops carrot seed oil (*Daucus carota*) essential oil
5 drops lemon verbena (*Lippia citriodora*) essential oil
6 drops rosemary verbenone (*Rosmarinus officinalis, verbenone type*) essential oil
4 drops lavender (*Lavandula vera*) essential oil
⅓ ounce avocado oil
⅓ ounce evening primrose oil

2-ounce glass bottle

Pour hazelnut oil in bottle. Add essential oils, close bottle, and roll between your palms to disperse the oils. Top off with avocado and evening primrose oils, close bottle, and agitate a second time.

Cleanse and tone skin. Apply 3 or 4 drops to a cotton pad or fingertips and wipe over entire face. To plump up the skin, use serum in conjunction with facial massage (see page 84).

SKIN PERSONALITY

SR   ER

MAKES 2 OUNCES

PREP TIME:
20 MINUTES

ROSEMARY ACNE SERUM

If you have oily or acne-prone skin, you may worry about putting oil on your skin. But what you may not realize is that oil actually removes oil. Furthermore, the two base oils used in this recipe, HAZELNUT and APRICOT KERNEL, are two of the lightest-weight astringent oils. TEA TREE OIL helps to break down hardened sebum and is well known for its strong antibacterial qualities. ROSEMARY, a strong skin-cell-regenerating oil, combines nicely with the toning properties of LEMON and JUNIPER.

1 ounce hazelnut oil
6 drops rosemary verbenone (*Rosmarinus officinalis, verbenone type*) essential oil
5 drops juniper (*Juniperus communis*) essential oil
5 drops tea tree (*Melaleuca alternifolia*) essential oil
4 drops lemon (*Citrus limonum*) essential oil
1 ounce apricot kernel oil

2-ounce glass bottle

Pour hazelnut oil in bottle. Add essential oils, close bottle, and roll between palms to disperse the oils. Top off with apricot kernel oil, close bottle, and agitate a second time.

Cleanse and tone skin. Apply 3 or 4 drops to a cotton pad or fingertips and wipe over entire face. To plump up the skin, use serum in conjunction with facial massage (see page 84).

GERANIUM REGENERATING SERUM

Mature skin is thinner than the skin of younger people and often lacks sufficient moisture. The combination of vegetal oils in this serum results in the highest possible percentage of GLA, an essential fatty acid in collagen synthesis, to make the skin firmer. The GERANIUM bouquet provides a sumptuous feel but the heart of this serum is the EVERLASTING. Also called IMMORTELLE, EVERLASTING earns its reputation by keeping skin looking younger. A potent anti-inflammatory herb, it helps remedy broken capillaries, soothe dry skin, and assist in cellular repair.

SKIN PERSONALITY

MAKES 2 OUNCES

PREP TIME:
20 MINUTES

1 ounce hazelnut or apricot kernel oil
4 drops everlasting (*Helichrysum italicum*) essential oil
6 drops geranium (*Pelargonium odorantissimum*) essential oil
4 drops frankincense (*Boswellia carterii*) essential oil
3 drops chamomile (*Anthemis nobilis*) essential oil
⅓ ounce rose hip seed oil
⅓ ounce evening primrose oil
⅓ ounce avocado oil

2-ounce glass bottle

Pour hazelnut oil into bottle. Add essential oils, close bottle, and roll between palms to disperse the oils. Top off with rose hip seed oil, evening primrose oil, and avocado oil, close bottle, and agitate a second time.

Cleanse and tone skin. Apply 3 or 4 drops to a cotton pad or fingertips and wipe over entire face. To plump up the skin, use serum in conjunction with facial massage (see page 84).

Contrary to popular belief among estheti-cians, massage does not damage the protein collagen, whose strong white fibers are stronger than steel wire of the same weight. In fact, massage is beneficial to the skin in many ways. First, it stimulates blood circulation to the tissues, increasing the supply of nutrients and oxygen. Second, the increased circulatory flow creates heat, which allows the essential oils to penetrate the skin more easily. Massage also relaxes the superficial and deep facial muscles—of which there are over thirty. When these muscles become tight, they constrict the blood flow and the supply of vital nutrients that feed the skin.

TO GIVE YOURSELF A FACIAL MASSAGE, start with a lavender compress. Compresses are relaxing moist-heat treatments that increase local circulation to improve dull facial com-plexion. Fill the bathroom sink with warm water. Add 2 or 3 drops of lavender (*Lavandula vera*) essential oil and swish water around to disperse the oil. Soak a washcloth in water, wring out, and apply to face. Inhale deeply to receive relaxing benefits.

Apply serum to fingertips and rub hands together to warm the oil. Gently press oil on to the face beginning at the chin and working up the face toward the hairline. At the center of the forehead make small, circular movements, sweeping outward toward temples. Repeat the same circular stroke beginning on either side of nose and move laterally to massage cheeks, jaw-line, and chin. Follow by stimulating the facial reflex points as directed to increase energy flow.

FACIAL REFLEX POINTS

Press and hold each point for 5 seconds using medium pressure.

1. Using thumbs, press down at the supraor-bital notch at inside of each eyebrow on either side of the nose. Finish by gliding thumbs outward across eyebrow.

2. Using index fingers, press down at the out-side edge of the eyebrow.

3. Using index finger, press down on either side of nose, below orbital bone just below pupil of eye.

4. Using index finger, repeat ¼ inch below last reflex point on either side of nose.

5. Repeat again, ¼ inch below last reflex point on either side of nose.

6. Using index finger, gently press on TMJ joint (temporomandibular joint) of jaw.

Finish treatment with a second lavender com-press to increase absorption of essential oils.

MASKS

The purpose of a mask is to **recharge** your skin, by either adding more moisture, exfoliating dead skin cells, or clearing away excess oil. Applying a mask is also a good opportunity to give the skin a dose of vitamins, antioxidants, and essential fatty acids, especially if you have been on the run and haven't been eating right or maintaining a proper skin-care regimen.

AVOCADO HONEY MASK

There is a reason every skin-care book has a recipe for an avocado mask: this fruit is simply so rich in **proteins, vitamins, lecithin,** and **essential fatty acids** that it is like a well-balanced meal for the skin. This avocado mask will leave your skin **smooth** and **soft.** If you want to add extra moisture to the mask, include the COCONUT OIL, which is high in saturated fats.

SKIN PERSONALITY

MAKES ½ CUP

PREP TIME:
10 MINUTES

    ½ avocado, peeled and pitted
    1 egg
    1 tablespoon plain yogurt
    1 teaspoon baking soda
    1 tablespoon coconut oil (optional)

Combine all ingredients in a blender and process for 30 seconds. Apply immediately to clean skin and leave on for 5 to 10 minutes. Rinse off with warm water.

PURIFYING GREEN TEA MASK

SKIN PERSONALITY

HR

MAKES ½ CUPS

PREP TIME:
10 MINUTES

Clays are traditionally used in skin care for their drawing properties—as they dry they **pull out excess oil** and **dirt** and leave the skin feeling clean. This mask uses KAOLIN CLAY and BENTONITE CLAY, which are sold at health-food and specialty stores.

1 teaspoon green tea infusion (see page 69)
2 teaspoons aloe vera gel
1 teaspoon honey
1½ tablespoons kaolin clay
½ tablespoon bentonite clay
2 drops rosemary (*Rosmarinus verbenone*) essential oil
1 drop lavender (*Lavandula vera*) essential oil

Combine green tea infusion, aloe vera gel, and honey in mixing bowl and stir well. Slowly sprinkle in the kaolin and bentonite clays while stirring. Add the essential oils and combine well. Apply to clean face immediately and leave on for 10 minutes. Rinse off with warm water.

eye care

The eye area seems to be the first place that women notice the signs of aging. Fine lines begin to appear around the eyes in the late thirties and early forties, and under-eye puffiness becomes more of a regular occurrence. Seasonal allergies as well as food sensitivities can also cause eyes to swell.

A **CHAMOMILE COMPRESS** is the perfect ammunition to use to fight puffiness after a late night on the town or to use on a daily basis to soothe tired, puffy eyes. The anti-inflammatory properties of chamomile help to calm swollen tissue. Place 2 chamomile tea bags in a small bowl and cover with ¼ cup boiling water. Let cool. Place in refrigerator. When you're ready to apply the compress, squeeze excess fluid from tea bags and place over eyes. For added comfort, wrap an eye pillow in plastic wrap to prevent tea bags from staining it and place over tea bags on eyes to relax entire eye area.

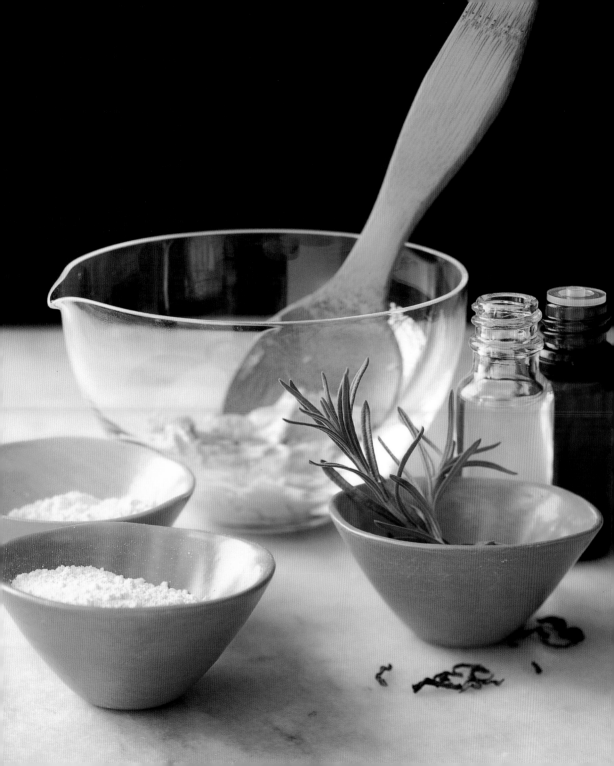

HAND CARE

The hand is a fascinating appendage, a small peninsula of flesh and bone that is a loyal servant, carrying out our most basic needs and desires: dialing a phone number, opening a door, eating an apple, caressing a lover. If you are like me, your hands also receive a fair amount of abuse. They fidget and wring, pull weeds, wash dishes, and do hundreds of other tasks. Add to that exposure to the elements and our hands may not be a very pretty sight.

The good news is that there are many nourishing rituals and recipes for the hands, which are usually very forgiving when treated properly.

HAND SOAK

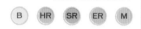

SKIN PERSONALITY

MAKES 2¼ CUPS

PREP TIME:
2 MINUTES

Begin your repentance by doing a hand soak.

2 cups warm water
1 tablespoon milk
1 teaspoon baking soda
3 drops tea tree *(Melaleuca alternifolia)* essential oil
1 tablespoons lemon juice (optional)
2 tablespoons white wine vinegar (optional)

Put the warm water in a bowl and add the milk and baking soda. Soak hands for 5 minutes to soften cuticles. (If cuticles are ragged and sore, add the tea tree oil to facilitate the healing process.)

Remove hands from bath and dry them. Clip and file nails and push back any cuticles that are in need of maintenance. If any of the nails are discolored, soak them again, but this time with the lemon juice and white wine vinegar.

HAND SOFTENER

This rich softener is fortified with creamy ALMOND and AVOCADO OILS to deeply penetrate the skin and organic BEESWAX to seal in moisture. The fresh LEMON VERBENA scent is hypnotic. Use it with the **HAND MASSAGE** (sidebar) for a luxurious experience.

1½ teaspoons shea butter
1 teaspoon beeswax
1 tablespoon lecithin
1 teaspoon sweet almond oil
1 teaspoon avocado oil
2 tablespoons lemon balm infusion (see page 69)
8 drops lemon verbena (*Lippia citriodora*) essential oil
2 drops lavender (*Lavandula angustifolia*) essential oil

2-ounce jar

Place cosmetic jar in a saucepan filled with water and gently boil for 5 minutes to sterilize jar. Melt the shea butter, beeswax, lecithin, sweet almond oil, and avocado oil in a double boiler or in a heat-proof measuring cup set in a pan of simmering water. In a separate pan, heat the lemon balm infusion until almost boiling and then slowly add it to the oil-and-wax mixture while beating with a whisk. Remove from heat. Stir in essential oils as mixture begins to cool but before it sets. Pour into a sterile jar. Keep refrigerated to discourage spoiling.

NOTE: Lecithin is available at many health food stores.

SKIN PERSONALITY

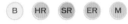

MAKES 2 OUNCES

PREP TIME:
45 MINUTES

hand massage

Apply a small amount of hand softener to back of hand and gently squeeze fingers. Using small circular thumb movements, trace four parallel lines on palm of hand beginning at the base of hand and working toward fingers. Massage each finger, gently pulling on it to relax the joint. Finish by squeezing the fleshy web between the thumb and index finger. Repeat on other hand. Cover with cotton gloves to increase hydration.

FOOT CARE

There are more than 250,000 sweat glands in the soles of the feet. So when they're confined to the airtight humidor of our shoes all day it's no wonder our feet look the way they do. These next recipes will provide your feet with a little TLC to bring them back to life.

NAIL FUNGUS RELIEF

SKIN PERSONALITY

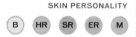

MAKES ½ OUNCE

PREP TIME:
20 MINUTES

This is an effective remedy for unsightly yellow toenail fungus, although TEA TREE OIL, the standard cure-all for nail fungus, may not be strong enough if the fungus has been allowed to grow unhindered for some time. This recipe combines the powerful antiseptic action of three phenol-type essential oils: THYME, TEA TREE, and OREGANO.

½ ounce sweet almond oil
30 drops thyme (*Thymus vulgaris*, thymol type) essential oil
15 drops oregano (*Origanum vulgaris*) essential oil
15 drops tea tree (*Melaleuca alternifolia*) essential oil

½ ounce glass bottle

Fill bottle halfway with sweet almond oil. Add essential oils, close bottle, and shake well. Top off with remaining sweet almond oil, close bottle, and agitate again. Apply to affected area 2 times a day. Discontinue use after 1 month if you see no signs of improvement.

PEPPERMINT FOOT BATH

The restorative hot foot bath is a popular naturopathic technique to draw blood away from the head and extremities in order to release toxins and ease stress (this technique is a very effective natural remedy for getting rid of headaches by drawing excess blood from the head to the feet).

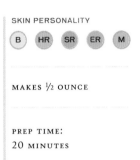

SKIN PERSONALITY

B HR SR ER M

MAKES ½ OUNCE

PREP TIME:
20 MINUTES

> 1 teaspoon sweet almond oil
> 3 drops peppermint (*Mentha piperita*) essential oil

Fill a large bowl or tub with warm water and add the sweet almond oil and the peppermint essential oil. Swish with your hand to disperse oils. Place feet in bath and soak for 5 to 10 minutes until your feet feel cool and tingly. For extra stimulation, place some pebbles or marbles in the tub and roll your feet back and forth over them.

ROSEMARY MINT FOOT SCRUB

Remove dry, calloused skin with this stimulating exfoliating paste.

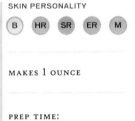

SKIN PERSONALITY

B HR SR ER M

MAKES 1 OUNCE

PREP TIME:
10 MINUTES

> 1 ounce sweet almond oil
> 3 drops rosemary (*Rosmarinus officinalis*) essential oil
> 3 drops peppermint (*Mentha piperita*) essential oil
> ½ cup cornmeal

Combine sweet almond oil with rosemary and peppermint essential oils in a bowl. Slowly stir in cornmeal until it becomes a thick paste. Apply to soles of the feet in a circular scrubbing motion, giving extra attention to callus-prone heels and toes.

NOTE: For extra-calloused feet use sea salt instead of cornmeal, for deeper exfoliation.

TEA TREE AND LEMON FOOT BALM

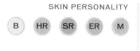

SKIN PERSONALITY

(B) (HR) (SR) (ER) (M)

MAKES 2 OUNCES

PREP TIME:
45 MINUTES

1½ teaspoons shea butter

1 teaspoon grated beeswax

1 tablespoon lecithin

1 teaspoon sweet almond oil

1 teaspoon avocado oil

2 tablespoons lemon balm infusion (see page 69)

8 drops tea tree (*Melaleuca alternifolia*) essential oil

6 drops lemon (*Citrus limonum*) essential oil

2-ounce glass jar

foot massage

1. Apply a small amount of foot balm to palms and rub palms together to coat hands evenly. Support the left ankle on your right knee. Place both hands on foot with fingers on top and thumbs below foot. Using firm pressure, wring the foot with your hands.

2. Continue to rest your left ankle on your right knee. Using your thumb, work on the instep, or inside, of the foot. Begin at the heel and, using small circular strokes, work alongside the bone up to the big toe.

3. Sink your thumb into any tender areas that might need extra attention.

4. Finish by massaging the top of the foot. Work each toe separately. Using your thumb, work the fleshy areas between the bones beginning at the toes and working toward the ankle. Repeat on opposite foot. Put on cotton socks to retain hydration.

Place cosmetic jar in a saucepan filled with water and gently boil for 5 minutes to sterilize jar. Melt the shea butter, beeswax, lecithin, sweet almond oil, and avocado oil in a double boiler or in a heat-proof measuring cup set in a pan of simmering water. In a separate pan, heat the lemon balm infusion until almost boiling and then slowly add it to the oil-and-wax mixture while beating with a whisk. Remove from heat. Add essential oils as mixture begins to cool but before it sets. Pour into jar and use for a foot massage (sidebar). Keep refrigerated to discourage spoiling.

NOTE: Lecithin is available at many health food stores.

BODY BASICS

There is something so satisfying about making your own body oils, lotions, and scrubs. It's not about saving money; rather it is a chance to tap into our inner alchemist and indulge in the home spa experience. You just won't know what you can create until you roll up your sleeves and get messy.

ALMOND PASTE BODY SCRUB

The sweet, luscious almond bouquet is so intoxicating that you will be tempted to eat this scrub (but don't—unless you are feeling the need to exfoliate your esophagus). SWEET ALMOND OIL is rich in essential fatty acids and therefore prized for its hydrating and emollient properties.

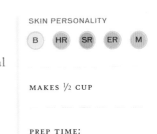

SKIN PERSONALITY

B   HR   SR   ER   M

MAKES ½ CUP

PREP TIME:
20 MINUTES

2 tablespoons sweet almond oil
1 tablespoon coconut oil
1 tablespoon baking soda
1 teaspoon aloe vera gel
¼ teaspoon vanilla extract
½ cup ground almonds

Place the sweet almond and coconut oils, baking soda, aloe vera gel, and vanilla extract in a blender and puree until smooth. Add the almonds and blend on low speed for 60 seconds. While skin is damp, apply to liberally to areas of dry, flaky skin. Let skin absorb almond paste for several minutes, and then rinse off with warm water.

JAVANESE MILK BATH TREATMENT

SKIN PERSONALITY

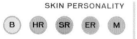

MAKES 1 CUP

PREP TIME:
10 MINUTES

Milk is used for **bathing** in many cultures because of its hydrating, **softening** properties and luxurious feel. This recipe combines milk with the **exotic fragrances** of the South Pacific—YLANG-YLANG, SANDALWOOD, and VANILLA.

1 cup whole milk
1 tablespoon baking soda
1 teaspoon honey
1 teaspoon vanilla extract
4 drops ylang-ylang *(Cananga odorata)* essential oil
6 drops sandalwood *(Santalum album)* essential oil
3 drops jasmine *(Jasminum grandiflorum)* essential oil

In a small pan, heat the milk, baking soda, honey, and vanilla extract over low heat until warm. Remove from heat and add essential oils. Stir with spoon and pour into bathwater.

NOTE: Use the ALMOND PASTE BODY SCRUB (see page 93) with this treatment in the bath for a complete Indonesian experience.

WINTER LEGS MASK

SKIN PERSONALITY

MAKES ½ CUP

PREP TIME:
10 MINUTES

When you find your legs looking like the Creature from the Black Lagoon, it's time to give them a **moisture surge.** This treatment is good to do after a body scrub once the dry skin has been removed.

1 avocado, peeled and pitted
1 tablespoon plain yogurt
1 tablespoon shea butter
1 teaspoon baking soda

Combine all of the ingredients in a blender and puree on low speed for 30 seconds.

In the bathtub, apply a thick layer to your legs, propping them up on the ledge of the tub for 5 minutes while mask absorbs. Rinse off with warm water.

HONEY VANILLA LIP BALM

This **soothing** balm combines the protective properties of BEESWAX with the rich texture of HONEY, to relieve chapped or cracked lips. The anti-inflammatory CALENDULA **protects** your lips against the elements. And the heavenly **aroma** of VANILLA makes this delicious treatment irresistible.

SKIN PERSONALITY

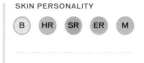

MAKES ½ OUNCE

PREP TIME:
45 MINUTES

½ ounce Calendula Infused Oil (see page 67)
½ tablespoon grated beeswax
5 drops vanilla (*Vanilla planifolia*) essential oil
1 tablespoon honey

½-ounce glass ointment jar

Place ointment jar in a saucepan filled with water and gently boil for 5 minutes to sterilize jar. Place calendula-infused oil and beeswax in a heatproof glass measuring cup, and set cup in a shallow pan of simmering water. Heat, stirring constantly, until all of the ingredients are melted. Remove from heat, add vanilla essential oil and honey, and stir until combined. Pour into ointment jar and place in the refrigerator to set.

Apply to lips whenever they need extra protection.

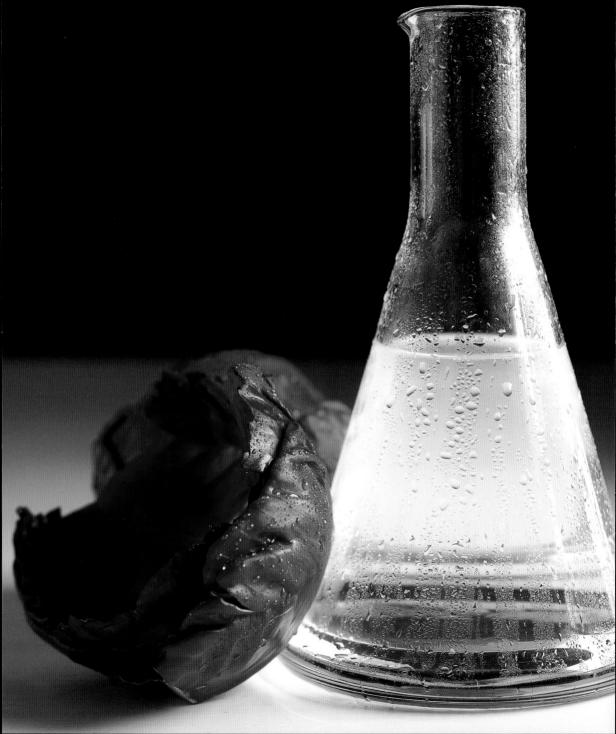

detox and retox

EATING FOR BEAUTIFUL SKIN

3

We all have our own relationship with eating. As for myself, I have come to forgive my excesses and, in fact, accept them if I can see them in the larger context of a generally healthy diet. My credo, **"Everything in moderation—even moderation,"** speaks to the inevitability of eating cassoulet or an apple butterscotch tart but puts such indulgences in perspective: balancing cheese and dessert with an overall diet of healthy foods and eating habits.

Our diet has a great deal to do with how we look and feel. Unfortunately, too often we eat convenience foods in order to save time. These empty foods wreak havoc on our bodies, since they are commonly loaded with some of the least healthful ingredients: sugar, white flour, hydrogenated fats, additives, and preservatives. And while the body automatically rids itself of many toxins, excessive processed foods, pesticides, food additives, alcohol, drugs, and a host of internal factors such as stress and toxic emotions can interrupt the body's natural detoxification process. When excess toxins build up in the body, inflammatory responses such as eczema, psoriasis, and skin infections can appear. By cleansing the body of some of these irritants, we can dramatically improve the clarity, texture, and appearance of our skin.

My aim in this chapter is to show you what the most harmful foods are for your skin, the right foods to eat, and a detox plan for those times when, despite our best intentions, we overindulge in the wrong things.

EATING WELL

If there is one place I am useless in restraint, it is around the dining room table, as no excuse is ever needed for indulging in good food and wine. I enjoy the gift of appetite, especially when paired with the company of friends.

Unfortunately, we live in a society that has a love-hate relationship with food. On the one hand obesity and overeating are epidemic in America; on the other a pervasive psychology of deprivation dominates the fashion, beauty, and fitness industries. But these attitudes regarding food don't take into account the most important (and simple) beauty secret of all: don't eat junk. Eating well means forgetting about watching calories and grams of fat and instead eating unprocessed foods that are full of flavor, have plenty of nutritional value, and support the earth's sustainability. It means abandoning "fat free" foods and embracing health.

The essence of the Slow Food Movement is to take the time to enjoy locally grown food and ingredients as opposed to grabbing a hamburger at a fast-food restaurant. Think of a dinner with fresh fish, vegetables from a local farm, and a glass of wine from a local vineyard. In my opinion, it doesn't get better than this, but Big Food and the agribusiness have other interest in mind, mainly getting a uniform food product to your table as fast as possible. Basically this means using lots of pesticides or in some cases genetically engineered, pest-resistant seeds and cultivating the land in such a way as to obtain the highest yield per acre. If you have had a hard time recently finding a tomato or an ear of corn that actually has taste you have experienced this process.

For the best skin-nourishing nutrients, choose organic foods whenever you can. In addition to their lack of potentially carcinogenic pesticides, organic foods have been shown to be higher in nutrients than conventionally grown foods. And anyone who has tended a garden can attest to the vibrancy and lushness of a just-picked cantaloupe or tomato. Fresh, organically grown plant material has a vibrational energy that nourishes the body right down to the cellular level. The hydrogenated, indefinitely preserved, prepackaged food that we see at our supermarket has almost none of the vitamins, nutrients, or vitality of the plant material from which it came.

DESTRUCTIVE FOODS

There are some food ingredients whose effects on the body make us feel bad physiologically as well as emotionally by triggering cravings and profound chemical changes in the body. The most destructive of these changes to skin health is the inflammatory response that the body develops to combat irritants. To prevent this inflammatory response, stick to low-glycemic foods. These are foods that do not rapidly convert to sugar, the most destructive inflammatory agent. High-glycemic foods include pasta, desserts, candy, juices, high-starch vegetables like potatoes and corn, and cereals such as cornflakes. To learn more about foods that are high on the glycemic index visit www.glycemicindex.com.

My advice is to know thy enemy and indulge in the foods discussed below only occasionally.

SUGAR

Sugar causes inflammation in several ways. When blood sugar goes up, it creates free radicals that attack our body on a cellular level by oxidizing fats. These oxidized fats convert to a chemical compound called aldehydes that trigger an inflammatory response. Sugar is bad for just about every system in the body, including the immune system, the cardiovascular system, and especially the skin, by breaking down the lipid barriers of the cells. Try an herbal remedy called stevia, available at health food stores, to sweeten your beverages naturally. Stevia is three hundred times sweeter than sugar but does not have its harmful side effects.

REFINED FLOUR

Refined flours used in foods such as pasta and breads are high-glycemic starches that act like sugars. Whole grains, on the other hand, are made up of the health-enhancing bran (the outer layer) and germ (the internal seed), which have fiber as well as nutritive phytochemicals. Several studies have documented that people who consume plenty of whole grains live longer than those who eat lots of refined flour.

HYDROGENATED FATS

Also known as trans-fatty acids, hydrogenated fats are added to many fast foods and packaged goods to extend their shelf life. These fats wreak havoc on the body by unleashing free radicals, which play a role in heart disease and cancer and cause a strong inflammatory response in the body.

ACID-FORMING FOODS

If you are eating carefully but your skin is persistently itchy or prone to rashes and other irritations, I recommend trying a pH kit available at health food stores. These easy-to-use kits will demonstrate the acidity or alkalinity in your body. If you have an elevated acidity level, avoid acid-forming foods such as coffee, alcohol, processed foods, and saturated fats from dairy and red meat, which can aggravate skin disturbances. Eat a more alkaline diet of grains, fruits, and vegetables, especially if you have a stress-reactive or environment-reactive skin personality.

FOOD ALLERGIES

Many people are allergic to common foods such as wheat, corn, soybeans, and dairy products. Removing problem foods from your diet can dramatically improve chronic skin conditions such as eczema and psoriasis. Keep a food journal, writing down everything you eat and how you feel one hour afterward for seven days. Include meals, snacks, and drinks. Observe and jot down any fluctuations in your energy level or symptoms such as headaches, muscle pain, or nasal congestion after eating certain foods. Most important, note how your skin changes: when do you see dryness, breakouts, puffiness, or rashes? Over the course of seven days you should be able to determine if certain foods are irritants.

BEAUTY FOODS

The basic rule of eating well is to consume a wide variety of organic fresh fruits, vegetables, and whole grains (brown rice, couscous, quinoa, and barley, not refined white flour or white rice). If you are not a vegetarian, stick to organic beef and poultry (from animals that have been given only vegetarian feed) and boost your intake of oily fish.

PHYTONUTRIENTS AND ANTIOXIDANTS

To really improve your skin's fitness, increase your intake of phytonutrients and antioxidants. These chemical compounds help to clean up cellular damage caused by free radicals. This is easy to do by zeroing in on the colorful foods that host an abundance of these natural chemicals, featured on page 105.

ESSENTIAL FATTY ACIDS

Despite our society's collective fear of fat, there are some beneficial fats that our body and especially our skin need in order to be healthy. Essential fatty acids

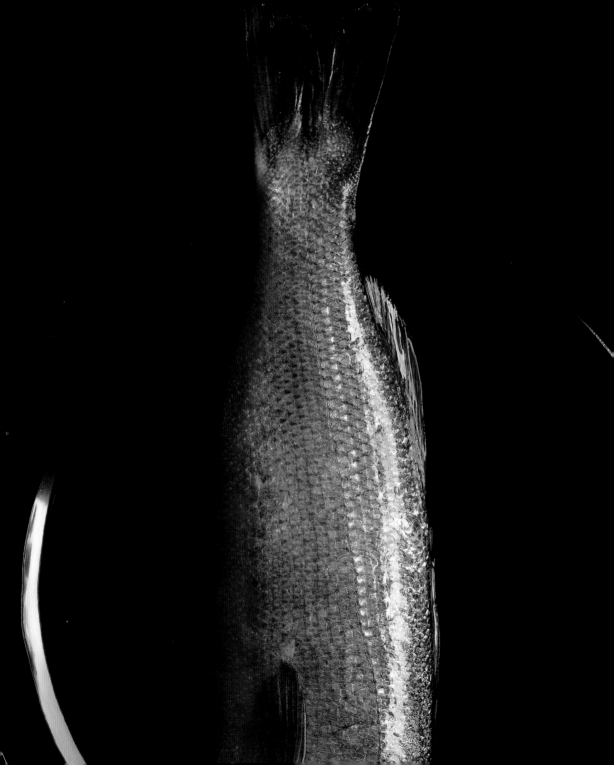

(EFAs), one of these beneficial fats, cannot be produced in the body and must be obtained through diet or supplements. EFAs come in two forms: omega-3 and omega-6. The omega-3s contain primarily alpha linoleic acid and the omega-6s contain linoleic acid and gamma linoleic acid. Linoleic acid helps skin cells maintain water as well as build dermal ceramides, which are the binding agents between skin cells that give them firmness and tonicity.

EFAs are converted to substances called prostaglandins, which act like hormones to help regulate several physiological functions, including maintenance of skin tone as well as cardiovascular health and fat metabolism. Stress, alcohol use, and a poor diet can block this conversion, so be sure to get enough EFA-containing foods in your diet.

EFAs are found in nonrefined oils primarily extracted from fish and plants. Cold-water fish such as sardines, cod, and salmon have a high concentration of EFAs. (Make sure that you eat wild salmon—avoid the farm-raised variety, which not only are loaded with antibiotics in order to help them endure captivity but also have high levels of PCBs, a carcinogenic chemical, due to the feed they ingest.) In the plant kingdom, flaxseed, evening primrose, black currant, and borage seed oil all contain alpha linoleic acid (the last three oils are beneficial when applied to the skin topically as well).

Make it easy to bring EFAs into your diet. Keep a bottle of flaxseed oil in your refrigerator and add a teaspoon to salad dressings. Or fill a peppermill with whole flaxseeds and grind them into soups, salads, or your favorite entrées. (Keep the peppermill in the fridge to keep the flaxseeds fresh.) Another way to get a boost of EFAs is to take 500 milligrams of black currant oil twice a day. Avoid fish oil capsules, which can be toxic and do not yield the same benefits.

FIBER

Eating foods that lack fiber or roughage leads to constipation. Constipation encourages toxicity since it increases the length of time waste products stays in the intestines. If these toxins are not expelled quickly they accumulate and may be absorbed into the intestines and bloodstream. They may also end up being excreted through different channels of the body, for example in mucus via the respiratory system or, in small amounts, through sweat in the skin, leading to skin imbalances.

Many of us find it difficult to maintain the recommended fiber intake of 25 to 30 grams a day. If you don't get that much fiber through you daily meals, supplement with psyllium husks (see page 133).

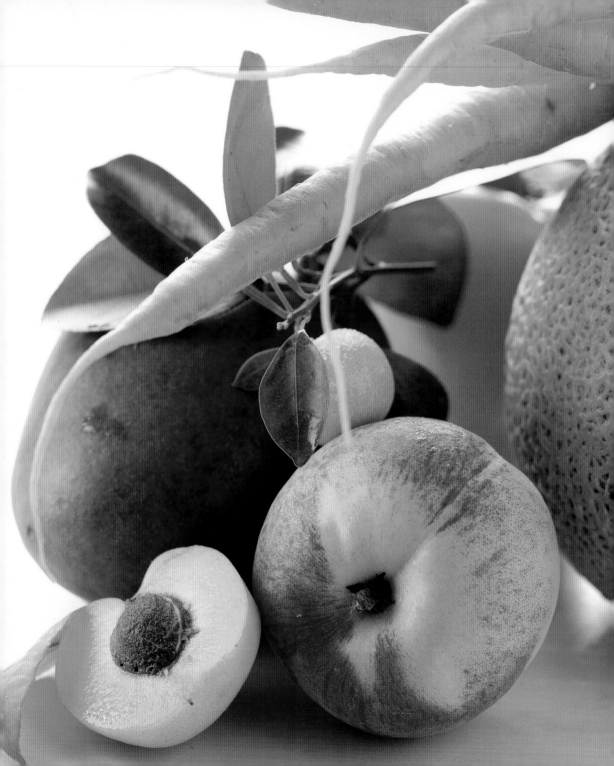

COLOR	BEST FOOD SOURCE	INTERNAL BENEFIT	BEAUTY TIP
RED	tomatoes, red peppers, beets, strawberries, grapes, wine, raspberries, watermelon, cherries	**LYCOPENE**, a carotenoid that is a potent free radical scavenger	Pack a container of strawberries, raspberries, or grapes to snack on at work. Enjoy a glass of organic red wine with dinner.
ORANGE	cantaloupe, oranges, mangoes, papayas, apricots, grapefruit, carrots, orange peppers, sweet potatoes	**ALPHA-CAROTENE** and **BETA-CAROTENE**, which protect the skin from UV free-radical and DNA damage	Nibble on raw carrots throughout the day or dip carrots or pepper slices in hummus for a high-protein lunch.
YELLOW	corn, squash, yellow peppers, bananas, nectarines	**BETA CRYPTOTHANXIN**, which helps intracellular communication	Eat a banana once a day.
GREEN	spinach, avocados, kale, broccoli, Brussels sprouts, pears, apples, grapes, green tea	**VITAMIN E**, necessary for the growth of human tissue; **CAROTENOIDS** and **FLAVONOIDS**, which provide antioxidant benefits	Drink 5 cups of green tea daily.
PURPLE	eggplant, plums, grapes, blueberries	**ANTHOCYANINS**, which delay cellular aging	Spread plum preserves on your toast at breakfast and snack on baba ghanoush (eggplant pâté) spread on crackers.

beauty foods

SKIN FOOD SHOPPING LIST

The first step to getting yourself on the path to eating well and nourishing your skin is to fill your kitchen with healthful food options. Begin by cleaning out your cupboards and refrigerator, throwing away any processed, nutrient-poor foods that may tempt you. Most important, throw away all "fat-free" convenience foods. The foods below are all low on the glycemic index. Make copies of the shopping list that follows and use it as a template for shopping each time you go to the grocery store.

shopping list

WHOLE GRAINS AND NUTS
__ Almonds
__ Barley
__ Brown rice
__ Cashews
__ Couscous
__ Flaxseeds
__ Oatmeal
__ Pine nuts
__ Pita bread
__ Sesame seeds
__ Whole wheat or barley flour bread
__ Whole wheat pasta

MEAT AND POULTRY
__ Organic beef
__ Organic free-range chicken
__ Organic free-range turkey

FISH
__ Albacore or bluefin tuna
__ Anchovies
__ Flounder
__ Mackerel
__ Sardines
__ Scallops
__ Sea bass
__ Sole
__ Trout
__ Wild Alaskan salmon

VEGETABLES
__ Asparagus
__ Avocados
__ Beans (black, kidney, lima)
__ Bell peppers (red, yellow, green)
__ Broccoli, broccoli rabe
__ Brussels sprouts
__ Cabbage
__ Cauliflower
__ Cucumber
__ Eggplant
__ Leafy greens (kale, Swiss chard)
__ Lettuce
__ Lentils
__ Mushrooms
__ Onions, garlic
__ Soybeans, tofu
__ Spinach
__ Tomatoes
__ Watercress

FRUIT
__ Apples
__ Berries (blueberries, strawberries, raspberries)
__ Grapefruit
__ Lemons, limes
__ Melons (cantaloupe, honeydew)
__ Oranges
__ Peaches
__ Pears
__ Plums

SNACK FOODS
__ Baba ghanoush
__ Cherry tomatoes
__ Hummus
__ Olives
__ Pumpkin or sunflower seeds
__ Rice or water crackers

DAIRY
__ Feta cheese
__ Hard cheese (Parmesan, manchego)
__ Organic eggs
__ Plain yogurt (with active cultures)

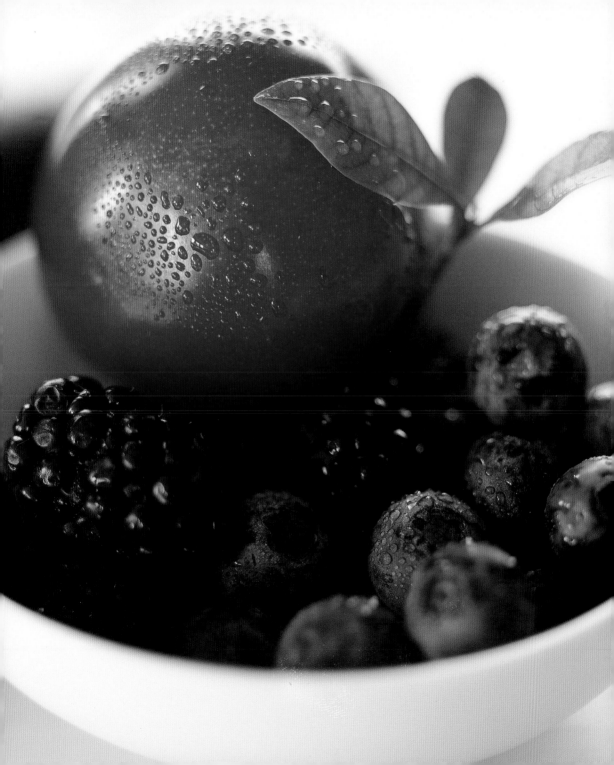

DETOX

Is it possible to love eating and yet still look and feel beautiful? I believe that the answer is yes. The dilemma I face when I flip through most health and well-being books is that these writers focus too heavily on the health-promoting benefits of their regimens and seem to forget about the sheer pleasure of food. Who wants to live that way? There's too much to enjoy. The Chilean novelist Isabel Allende writes, "I repent of my diets, the delicious dishes rejected out of vanity, as much as I lament the opportunities for making love that I let go by because of the pressing tasks or puritanical virtue."

So go ahead and enjoy yourself, indulge when you feel like it, and when things feel out of balance, rely on a detox program to get you on track with the right foods again. That way, when the inevitable retox comes—when we fill up on all the wrong things—you won't panic, you'll know what to do.

DETOX QUESTIONNAIRE

The skin is the largest organ of detoxification. Increasing numbers of people suffer from eczema, psoriasis, and skin infections that are an inflammatory response to the build up of toxins in the body. Complete the questionnaire to determine your need for detoxification. Rate the frequency with which you experience the symptoms on the facing page by tilling in the appropriate number for each.

FREQUENTLY	3
OCCASIONALLY	2
RARELY	1
NEVER	0

If you are experiencing any of the symptoms (see facing page) frequently or have average or below average vitality, you will benefit from a detox program. Keep your score so that you can redo the questionnaire after you have completed your detox program and rate your progress.

Fatigue or fluctuations in energy even after a good night's rest   _____

Headaches or migraines   _____

Stiff joints or muscle pains   _____

Irritability or mood swings   _____

Insomnia (inability to fall asleep or stay asleep)   _____

Lowered immunity; frequent colds or flus   _____

Sinus congestion, sensitivity to allergens, or asthma   _____

Inefficient digestion (gas, constipation, or loose stools)   _____

Overeating or compulsive eating   _____

Low tolerance to caffeine or alcohol   _____

Bloating after meals   _____

Prolonged use of antibiotics   _____

Skin imbalances including acne, eczema, and psoriasis   _____

Dry, dull, or flaky skin   _____

Thin, ridged, or split nails   _____

Dark circles under eyes, puffiness under eyes   _____

Coating on tongue, body odor, excess mucus, or bad breath   _____

Smoking   _____

Exposure to hazardous chemicals, chemotherapy, or radiation   _____

Excessive use of alcohol, drugs, or over-the-counter medicines   _____

TOTAL   _____

SCORING

0-5=HIGH VITALITY

6-15=GOOD VITALITY

16-30=AVERAGE VITALITY

31-50=LOW VITALITY

51-60=HIGH BURNOUT AND TOXICITY

FOURTEEN-DAY DETOX PLAN

The main goal of a detox program is to encourage the removal of toxins already in your system and to reduce the amount of new toxins you take in. The following nutritional medicine program introduces gentle, cleansing foods to increase the removal of toxins and then uses phytonutrient-rich foods to repair weak organs and tissues. This process is supported with herbal supplements, detox baths, and mind-body techniques for enhanced results.

WEEK ONE: REST AND CLEANSE

AVOID THE FOLLOWING: processed foods, fried foods, convenience foods, meats, sugar, alcohol, coffee, tea, soft drinks, and milk-based products. Substitute the following: steamed vegetables (especially colorful ones rich in plant nutrients, such as sweet potatoes, carrots, bell peppers, and dark-green, leafy vegetables); fiber-rich whole-grain foods (unprocessed brown rice, couscous, or quinoa); protein derived from tofu, eggs, or oily fish such as salmon or sardines (rich in amino acids); and enzyme-rich fruits such as papaya, pineapple, berries, apples, and pears. Experiment with some of the health-promoting food recipes on pages 115-119 to support your body during your detox program.

FOCUS NOT ONLY ON WHAT YOU EAT BUT ALSO ON HOW YOU INGEST YOUR FOOD:

Eat your largest meal in the middle of the day to allow proper assimilation.

Eat consciously and slowly: do not eat while watching TV or on the run.

Fast daily for at least twelve hours (e.g., 7:00 P.M. to 7:00 A.M.).

WEEK TWO: REPAIR AND RENEW

Continue nutritional program as detailed, adding more fruits and vegetables. Reintroduce white meat such as organic free-range chicken or turkey. Add more phytonutrient-rich foods such as cruciferous vegetables (e.g., broccoli, Brussels sprouts, and cabbage).

Most naturopathic doctors and herbalists believe that toxins build up in the fatty tissue of the body as well as in the joints. It is not uncommon during the course a detox program to feel worse for several days as these toxins are released into your system, to be flushed out. Headaches, neck or back pains, and joint stiffness are some of the common symptoms. Don't be tempted to reach for sugar, coffee, or junk food but instead increase the activation of your liver enzymes to remove the toxins by eating more proteins, fruits, and vegetables that contain the building blocks that your liver will use to make glutathione, an essential antioxidant. Also, drink plenty of water (8 to 12 glasses per day) to help flush toxins out of the system.

WEEKEND DETOX

Use this weekend detox as a tune-up to help you get back on track when you feel yourself starting to revert to your old unhealthy habits. Plan ahead by first shopping for the foods listed in the chart on the following pages.

Essential to any detox program is a cleansing of mind and body. Leave the TV off and don't bother with the newspaper—let the mind rest along with the body.

detox Rx

Supplement your Fourteen-Day Detox Plan with the following:

NUTRITIONAL MEDICINE: Drink 5 cups daily of antioxidant rich green tea, which contains phytochemicals that have antibacterial and anticancer properties. Try the Iced Fiji Green Tea recipe on page 139.

HERBAL MEDICINE: Add 20 to 30 drops of a tincture made from dandelion (see page 132), a powerful liver cleansing herb, to juice or green tea and drink twice a day to support proper digestive functioning. To cleanse the colon of accumulated toxic material, take 2 capsules of psyllium husks (see page 133) during the Fourteen-Day Detox Plan before bedtime each night, along with 16 ounces of water (make sure you drink a lot of water with psyllium husks to prevent constipation).

BATH WATER CURES: Twice a week, take the Detox Water Cure (see page 127), a stimulating herbal bath with hot water and detoxifying herbal extracts.

MIND-BODY DETOX: Nurture yourself more and develop simple rituals that support vibrant health. Surround yourself with books and magazines that encourage a healthy lifestyle. Remove all processed foods from kitchen cabinets and create a new collection of healthful meal ideas. And, since sleep is the most important restorative agent, follow the sleep tips on page 21 to ensure that you get a good night's rest every night.

	MEALS	**EXERCISE**	**HERBAL REMEDIES**
FRIDAY P.M.	DINNER: DETOX SOUP (SEE PAGE 115) Make ICED FIJI GREEN TEA SPRITZER (see page 139) for weekend beverage. Drink 1 liter of water during course of evening.	Rest. Go to bed early and get plenty of sleep to let your body recharge.	Take 2 psyllium husk capsules with 8 ounces of water before bedtime.
SATURDAY A.M.	BREAKFAST: Oatmeal sweetened with apple cider OR Two poached eggs over whole-grain toast Drink 1 liter of water during A.M. including 2 glasses of ICED FIJI GREEN TEA SPRITZER (see page 139).	Take a yoga or Pilates class and allow tension-bound muscles to rejuvenate.	On rising, drink a cup of hot water flavored with the juice of 1 lemon and a pinch of stevia (see page 100).
P.M.	LUNCH: Sardine Pâté OR CLEMENTINE AND WATERCRESS SALAD (see page 117) DINNER: BROILED SALMON WITH ORANGE MISO GLAZE and SAUTÉED SPINACH (see page 118–119) Drink 1 liter of water during course of afternoon.	Go for a brisk walk and surround yourself with the calming benefits of the outdoors.	Afternoon tea: Prepare and drink a pot of skin-clarifying COMPLEXION TEA (see page 137). Take 2 psyllium husk capsules with 8 ounces of water before bedtime.
SUNDAY A.M.	BREAKFAST: Smoothie with fresh, bioactive yogurt, juices, and enzyme-rich fruit such as blueberries or strawberries Drink 1 liter of water during A.M. including 2 glasses of ICED FIJI GREEN TEA SPRITZER	Try a new physical activity—go kayaking, take a martial arts class, or go on a nature walk.	Add 20 to 30 drops of herbal tincture with skin-clarifying herbs such as burdock, dandelion, and red clover to juice or tea. Repeat twice daily for 21 days.
P.M.	LUNCH: DETOX SOUP DINNER: SABA TERIYAKI (see page 119) with steamed broccoli Drink 1 liter of water including 2 glasses of ICED FIJI GREEN TEA SPRITZER (see page 139).	Try a yoga video at home and do 30 minutes of stretching.	Research a flower essence that is best for your skin personality (see page 140) and begin to take this remedy daily.

HOME SPA

Bedtime:
Try a **REST HERBAL BATH** (see page 128) to soothe away stress from workweek.

Start your day with a **CLARIFYING FACIAL SAUNA** (see page 74) to remove impurities.

Follow with a **CLEANSING FACIAL GOMAGE** (see page 73) to exfoliate dull skin.

Bedtime:
Try a **DETOX HERBAL BATH** (see page 128) to stimulate cleansing of lymphatic system.

Blend and apply your own **FACE SERUM** (see pages 80–83) and follow with a nourishing **FACE MASSAGE** (see page 84).

Wind down by doing a relaxing **FOOT MASSAGE** (see page 92).

MIND HEALING

Seek repose after dinner:
read a book, listen to music, or write a letter.

Upon waking, sit quietly and meditate for 20 minutes before getting out of bed.

Find an activity you enjoy that stills the mind, such as knitting or editing a photo album.

Take a few hours and immerse yourself in health and fitness magazines.

PROFESSIONAL CARE

Have a maintenance session with a chiropractor or acupuncturist after work.

If your budget allows for it, try a private yoga or Pilates lesson to get the extra guidance your body needs.

If your budget allows for it, book a professional holistic facial or Swedish massage to nourish your body from head to toe. Or try an energizing **FOOT MASSAGE** (see page 92).

If you belong to a gym, take a sauna or steam bath to stimulate the cleansing process (a perfect after-yoga activity).

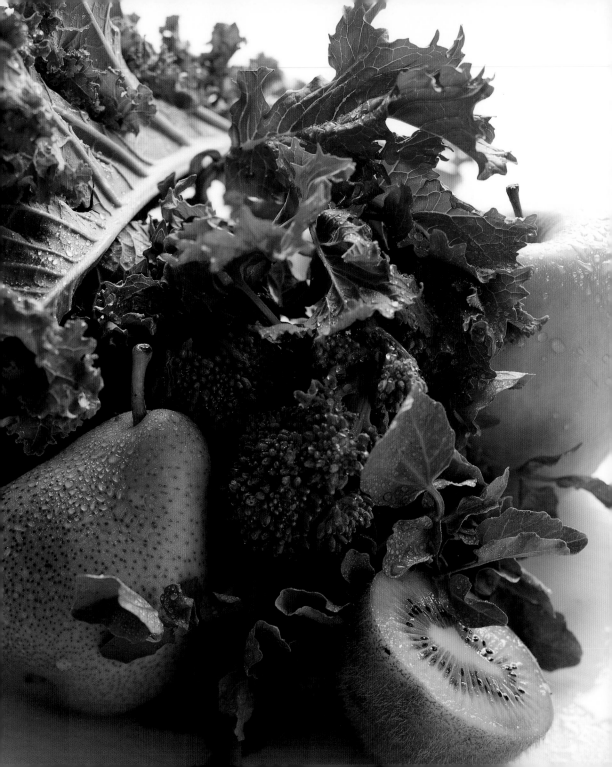

HEALING FOODS

Use the recipes that follow as an essential part of any detox plan, to restore your mind and body. These foods will help mitigate the effects of your latest binge without depriving you of the pleasure of eating delicious food.

DETOX SOUP

Miso, a flavorful paste made from fermented soybeans and grains, has several health benefits and can be found at any health food store or Asian grocery store. There are several varieties—soybean, rice, and barley—any of which can be used for this recipe. Traditionally served in Japan as a tonic for stomach or liver ailments, miso helps the body expel toxins and impurities.

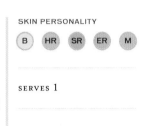

SKIN PERSONALITY

B · HR · SR · ER · M

SERVES 1

PREP TIME:
20 MINUTES

> 1 tablespoon miso paste
> 1 cup boiling water
> ½ cup soft tofu, cut into small pieces
> 2 scallions, thinly sliced
> A few watercress leaves (optional)
> Udon (optional)

Place the miso in a bowl. Add ¼ cup of the boiling water and stir to make a thin paste. Stir in the remaining water as well as all of the remaining ingredients. Serve immediately.

NOTE: WATERCRESS is an effective liver cleanser. UDON, a Japanese noodle, is sold at health food stores and Asian grocery stores.

SARDINE PÂTÉ

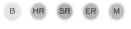

This pâté contains sardines and anchovies, both dark, oily fish rich in omega-3 fatty acids. It makes a quick and easy lunch or a tasty appetizer before a main meal.

SERVES 2

PREP TIME:
20 MINUTES

one 4-ounce can boneless sardines packed in water
2 anchovy fillets
1 small red onion, finely chopped
1 small clove garlic, minced
1 teaspoon white wine vinegar
1 tablespoon capers
1 tablespoon fresh flat-leaf parsley
1 tablespoon lemon juice

Combine all ingredients in a food processor and puree for 15 seconds. Serve with salad greens, rice, or rye crackers. Sprinkle with additional lemon juice, if desired.

CLEMENTINE AND WATERCRESS SALAD

WATERCRESS is a delicious sweet, spicy green that is grown in streambeds throughout North America. Its nutritious leaves contain calcium, magnesium, potassium, vitamin C, and beta-carotene and are an excellent blood purifier. WATERCRESS can lose its sweetness quite quickly once harvested so be sure to select the freshest watercress and avoid any plants with thick stems or flowers. The CLEMENTINES add an extra boost of vitamin C and beta-carotene.

SKIN PERSONALITY

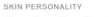
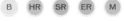

SERVES 2

PREP TIME:
20 MINUTES

1 small shallot
½ tablespoon champagne vinegar
1 tablespoon clementine juice
Salt
2 clementines
1 bunch watercress, washed and dried
1½ tablespoons extra-virgin olive oil

Mince the shallot and place in small bowl with vinegar, clementine juice, and a pinch of salt. Set aside. Peel clementines, separate into sections, and arrange on a bed of watercress. Drizzle olive oil into champagne-vinegar mixture while whisking briskly, and pour over salad. Add fresh-ground pepper to taste and toss well.

BROILED SALMON WITH ORANGE MISO GLAZE

SERVES 2

PREP TIME:
30 MINUTES

The omega-3 essential fatty acids found in oily fish such as SALMON contain potent anti-inflammatory compounds that help prevent free-radical damage. ORANGE JUICE contains vitamin C as well as beta-carotene to help protect the body. Think of this recipe as a rejuvenating booster.

3-inch piece ginger
2 tablespoons orange juice
2 tablespoons mirin
3 tablespoons miso
1 pound wild salmon fillet, skinned and halved
1 tablespoon extra-virgin olive oil
Salt

Preheat broiler.

Peel and grate ginger and over a small bowl squeeze pulp with hand to yield juice. Discard pulp and add ginger juice to orange juice, mirin, and miso. Mix well.

Brush top of salmon with olive oil, sprinkle with salt, and place in baking pan lined with aluminum foil. Place under broiler for 2 minutes. Remove from oven, turn fish over, and continue to broil for additional 2 minutes. Remove from oven, brush glaze onto fish, and return to oven to broil for 1 minute more. Serve with Sautéed Spinach (facing page).

SAUTÉED SPINACH

1 tablespoon extra-virgin olive oil
1 clove garlic, minced
1 pound fresh spinach leaves, washed thoroughly
Juice of ½ lemon
Salt

Heat oil in sauté pan or wok over medium heat. Add garlic, sauté briefly, and add spinach, stirring constantly until wilted (1 or 2 minutes). Add lemon juice and salt to taste, toss, and serve.

SABA TERIYAKI

Inexpensive and widely available, MACKEREL is one of the best sources of omega-3 essential fatty acids. The dark flesh of this fish combines beautifully with the pungent flavor of the teriyaki sauce.

2 tablespoons soy sauce
2 tablespoons sake or dry sherry
1 tablespoon mirin
1 teaspoon maple syrup
½ clove garlic, minced
1 scallion, minced
1 pound mackerel fillet, skinned and halved

Place soy sauce, sake, mirin, maple syrup, garlic, and scallion in a pan over medium-high heat and bring to a boil. Remove from heat and set aside. Heat a nonstick pan until very hot, add fish, and cook for 2 minutes over medium-high heat. Turn fish over, cover with marinade, and cook for 2 more minutes. Turn fish one more time, cook for 10 seconds, and remove from pan. Let sauce continue to cook until a thick, dark syrup emerges, about 1 minute. Spoon over fish and serve immediately.

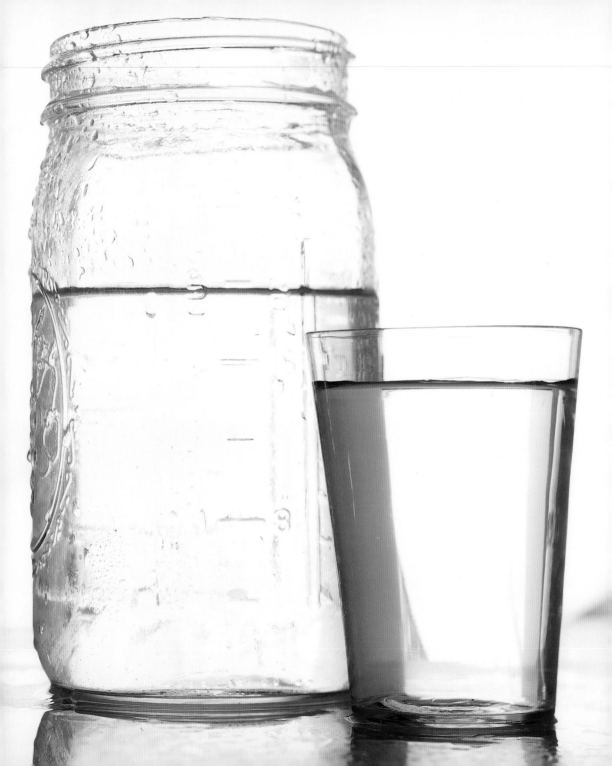

LIQUID REPLENISHMENT

Anyone concerned about the health of their skin knows that the recommended amount to consume is 2 to 3 liters per day. What is less clear is why drinking fluids is essential to skin health and the best way to consume them.

The reality about drinking enough liquids throughout the day is that there has to be a certain amount of vigilance involved. One of the questions I ask when I take a lifestyle history from a client at our spa is "Do you drink enough water?" and invariably the response is "not as much as I should." When I explain the benefits provided to the body by drinking plenty of liquid nourishment, I am often amused that many times the reason given for not drinking enough is the same: "But then I will have to pee!"

Exactly. Think of your kidneys as giant blood purifiers that use fluids to filter out the toxins and inflammatory agents in your body. The more you drink, the cleaner your system—and your skin—will be. When your urine is a pale yellow, you are ingesting enough water. When your urine is dark and cloudy, it's time to head to the water cooler.

Water is the best liquid replenishment there is, but much depends upon the type of water you are ingesting. Tap water is treated with chlorine to eliminate pathogens. However, chlorine is a harsh chemical that in a gaseous state is dangerous and unhealthful. Conventional drinking water may also contain industrial and agricultural contaminants that are best avoided. And lead from old pipes can show up in tap water and be hazardous as well.

Bottled water is better, but since you can't be sure that the water you are purchasing is not contaminated, the best bet is to purchase a water purifier for your home. This will ensure that the water you are ingesting does not contain toxic materials and will also save you the expense of buying bottled water.

Now comes the thornier issue of how to make sure you drink enough water. I find the best way is to consecrate a drinking vessel. My choice is a simple Ball Mason jar for two reasons. First, there is some evidence that plastic drinking bottles have the potential to leach chemicals into the water they hold, especially when subjected to sunlight or hot water. Second, a Mason jar has a measurement system written on the glass and you can see clearly how many ounces or milliliters you consume. Also, I find that a glass vessel does not impart a plastic taste and actually keeps the water cooler.

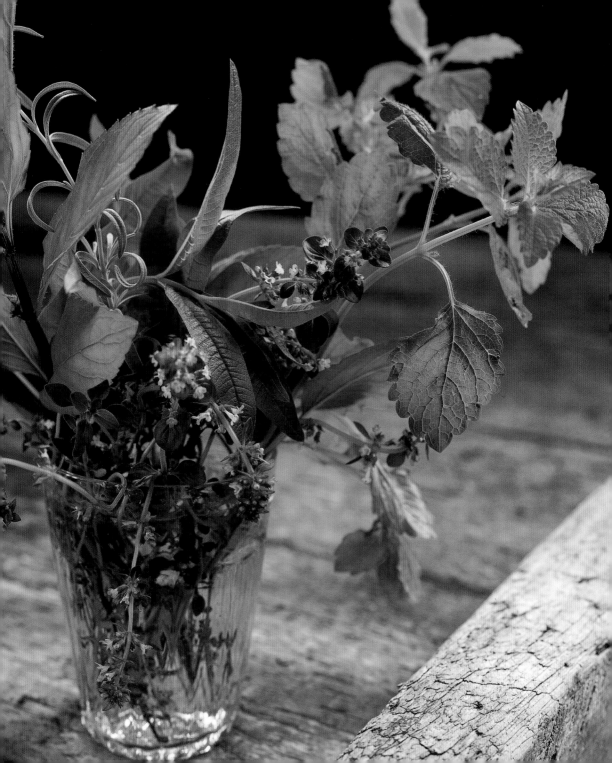

beauty in balance

RESTORATIVE
THERAPIES

RESTORATIVE THERAPIES

4

It seems that every beauty, health, and fitness magazine you read today keeps mentioning the word *balance*. To be honest, I am not really sure what they mean. When you think about it, balance is sort of an elusive concept really. To me it sounds like this nirvana-like plateau that if I tried to really discipline myself, I could attain. Maybe if I ate more soybean or drank less wine or took a yoga class every day, then maybe I'd be in that sort of Admiral's Club for balanced people. I'm not trying to be smart here. I think there are some people who probably are quite. . . . balanced. God bless them, they run the Iron Man marathons, eat only half their sandwich at lunch, and go to bed at a reasonable hour.

The *Oxford English Dictionary* defines balance as "to bring to or keep in equilibrium." The first part of that definition, "to bring to equilibrium," makes sense, but what about the second part? How does one keep, or maintain, equilibrium? In fact, you can't—to do so would defy the law of physics. Nature, of which we are a part, is all about cycles, ever changing, ebbing, flowing. So to expect ourselves to reach and maintain physical and emotional perfection is unrealistic.

The ups and downs are part of living, so it's important to have some strategies on hand for those low points when an acne flare-up arises, our energy is zapped, or we've overindulged in our vice of choice. In addition to our daily maintenance, practices such as massage, water cures, heat therapies, and energetic medicines such as homeopathy and flower essences can help rejuvenate the skin—not to mention bring relaxation and peace of mind when they're needed most.

So don't exhaust yourself trying to live in perfect balance—there's no such thing. Rather, accept that everyone cycles, and read this chapter to learn more about what you can do to turn things around when you're not feeling your best.

MASSAGE THERAPY

The renowned physician Avicenna (A.D. 980) recommended the "restorative friction" of massage for a variety of medicinal purposes. Likewise, doctors today recommend therapeutic massage for its physical and emotional benefits. Massage improves the circulation of blood and the movement of lymph fluids, reduces blood pressure, strengthens the immune system, relieves muscle pain, and aids relaxation of the entire body. But massage also enhances the health and nourishment of the skin. The kneading action of the flesh helps bring more oxygen and nutrients to the skin and at the same time encourages the removal of toxins. Massage also promotes the absorption of therapeutic essential oils as well as the hydration of the dermis with vitamin-rich vegetal oils. (Unfortunately, many massage therapists use the cheapest essential and vegetal oils they can find, which do not yield the benefits of high-quality ingredients.)

Although it may be more relaxing to receive a massage from a professional massage therapist, you can still experience the benefits of touch with a partner or through self-massage—and when you have a massage at home you can use the very best essential and vegetal oils. Essential oils can penetrate the tissues easily and enter the capillaries for quick distribution throughout the body. The most permeable areas of the body are the face, the soles of the feet, and the scalp.

Following the AROMATHERAPY BLENDING BASICS on page 64, create a massage oil blend that best fits your mood or is designed to treat a specific condition (you will need 1 ounce for a full body massage). Then ask a partner or a friend to give and/or receive a restorative massage. When you are giving a massage, begin by having your partner lie face up on the floor or bed. Pour the oil into your hands and wring them together to warm the oil. Place your hands over your partner's nose and have him or her take three deep, diaphragmatic breaths in order to stimulate the relaxation response. Then gently stroke, knead, and wring muscles of affected areas to release tension and revitalize the senses. Repeat once a week.

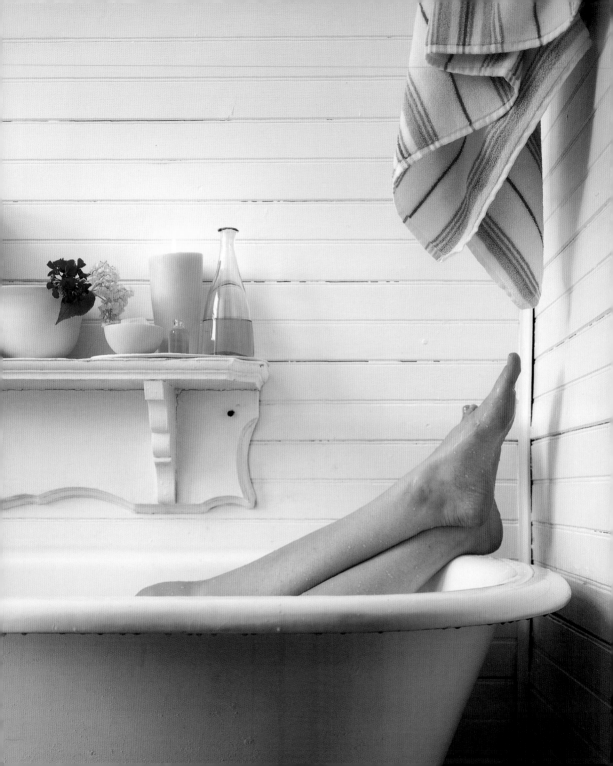

WATER CURES

Hydrotherapy is an important modality of natural healing. The therapeutic use of water, including alternating hot and cold water treatments (baths or showers), steam baths, inhalations, and compresses, strengthens the natural defenses of the body. Warm water is sedative, promotes perspiration, and acts as an analgesic and antispasmodic for muscles with stress-induced aches and pains. Hot water draws blood to the extremities. Cold water acts as a restorative tonic, boosting energy by bringing blood back to the heart. Alternating hot water with short bursts of cold water gets the blood and lymphatic fluid moving, pumping toxins out of the tissues.

Naturopathica water cures utilize the beneficial properties of the water along with the therapeutic properties of plant extracts and essential oils. Since essential oils are lipophilic, they try to escape from water and absorb into the fatty tissue of the skin and thus are more readily absorbed than through regular massage. Water cures are an excellent at-home follow-up treatment after a massage or spa visit.

There are three types of water cures: detox, rest, and renew. The therapeutic properties of the water cure depend upon three things: the temperature of the water, the length of time the body is immersed in the water, and the types of plant extracts used. These water cures are easy to do and will go a long way toward nourishing the principal healing systems of the body—the nervous, circulatory, lymphatic, and immune systems—all of which can affect the skin. See the AROMATHERAPY BLENDING BASICS on page 64 to learn how to incorporate these plant extracts into bath oils or shower gels.

SKIN BRUSHING

Skin brushing encourages the removal of dead skin cells and stimulates circulation, which in turn increases the removal of toxins. Purchase a vegetable brush with soft bristles, available at most health food stores, and rub a drop of a mild essential oil like lavender (*Lavandula vera*) on the brush to sterilize it. Using a light, sweeping stroke, begin at the feet and brush up the legs, front and back, toward the torso. To encourage the movement of lymph toward the main lymphatic ducts underneath the collarbones, always stroke toward the center of the body. Brush up both sides of the arms and across the shoulders, and continue up the back and neck. Finish the treatment using a clockwise spiral motion on the abdomen.

	BENEFITS	ESSENTIAL OILS	DURATION OF TREATMENT AND APPLICATION
DETOX HERBAL BATH	A stimulating bath to cleanse over-burdened digestive or lymphatic systems.	juniper lemon cypress grapefruit	Fill tub with hot water (100–110° F). Add 1 capful to still water and disperse with hand. Immerse body, 5-8 minutes max, until light perspiration appears. Towel off; rest for 5 minutes to let blood pressure normalize.
DETOX HERBAL SHOWER	Eases muscle soreness by flushing out lactic acid.	rosemary bay laurel basil	Add 1 teaspoon of oil or shower gel to damp washcloth and rub entire body briskly. Alternate hot and cold water (1 minute hot, 15 seconds cold). Repeat 3 times.
REST HERBAL BATH	A calming bath to ease stress related symptoms.	rose lavender mandarin neroli	Fill tub with warm water (92–100° F). Add 1 capful to still water and disperse with hand. Soak for 20-30 minutes.
RENEW HERBAL BATH	A revitalizing bath to combat fatigue or jet lag.	rosemary lavender grapefruit	Fill tub with cool or tepid water (80–92° F). Add 1 capful of bath oil to still water and disperse with hand. Soak in water for 10-15 minutes.

HEAT THERAPY

Sauna and steam treatments are another form of water cure and are among the most popular treatments in naturopathic medicine. Spending a few minutes in a sweltering sauna or steam room raises the heart rate, increasing circulatory flow to all of the organs of elimination including the liver, kidneys, and skin.

The obvious changes that the body experiences when exposed to heat are localized redness to the skin, vasodilatation, increased blood flow, rapid respiration, and perspiration. Perspiration eliminates by-products of cellular respiration, including sodium and some toxins. However, people with certain skin personalities, such as hormone reactive and environment reactive, may find heat therapies too stimulating for their skin and should therefore avoid intense heat.

The dry heat of the sauna is less intense than the wet heat of a steam bath, since steam is a more efficient conductor of heat than air is. Depending upon your tolerance of heat, you can stay in a sauna for up to 20 minutes. After that time the heat becomes oppressive to the circulatory system. For steam baths, a period of 10 minutes should be the maximum.

In Russia and Finland it is customary to have a friction massage when you take a sauna or steam bath. To partake of this stimulating ritual, as you begin to sweat apply 2 or 3 drops of rosemary essential oil to a soft natural-fiber brush or washcloth and gently rub the skin. This not only increases local circulation but also exfoliates.

Essential oils such as eucalyptus can be added to saunas and steam baths to enhance the respiratory benefits of a sauna or steam bath. However, because essential oils can be flammable, never place them directly on the hot rocks of a sauna; dilute them by adding 3 to 4 drops to a cup of water and then pour the fragrant water on the rocks.

For a quick deep cleansing of the face, try the Clarifying Facial Sauna on page 74 and follow with the fortifying Facial Massage on page 84 to give your skin a rosy glow.

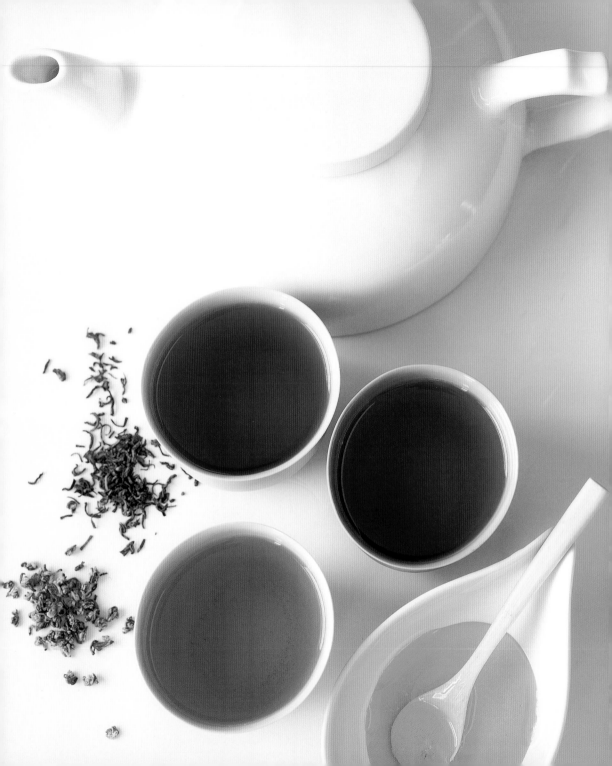

HERBAL SKIN-CARE PHARMACY

Herbal medicine is the oldest and most widely used form of health care in the world. Plants have played an important role in the history of medicine, and some of the world's greatest healing agents have been derived from the plant kingdom. Herbal remedies are still used throughout the world today. Many herbs have an enormous range of healing powers and can act as a restorative tonic to help the body function optimally.

Several herbs in particular are especially useful in skin care. Some are blood purifiers and diuretics and have a cleansing effect, some help to boost the immune system, and others heal skin conditions. They can be ingested internally in tea, liquid tincture, or capsule form. Externally, they can be applied to the skin as salves, oils, or ointments. You will definitely want to choose some of these remedies, depending upon your skin personality, to keep on hand. Either purchase them from a good health food or herbal remedy company (see Resources, page 142), or make some of these preparations yourself and enjoy participating in your own healing regimen.

	HERB	BENEFITS	APPLICATIONS	INSTRUCTIONS	PRECAUTIONS
skin-clarifying herbs	black currant	Skin-soothing herb rich in omega-6 fatty acid.	Take in capsule form.	Take 500 mg twice daily or as directed by physician to promote healthy skin.	None at recommended dose.
	burdock root *(Arctium lappa compositae)*	Blood purifier, rich in iron and minerals. Effective in treating dry and scaly skin disorders such as eczema or psoriasis.	Take in liquid tincture or capsule form alone or with other skin-clarifying herbs.	In tincture form, add 2 ml (50 drops) twice daily to juice or water. In capsule form, take 200 mg daily or as directed by physician.	Avoid during pregnancy and while nursing.
	calendula *(Calendula officinalis)*	Wound healer and skin soother.	Use externally in salve or ointment.	Apply to affected areas.	None.
	chamomile *(Matricaria chamomilla)*	Anti-inflammatory. Sedative and soothing to digestive system.	Apply externally to soothe skin. Drink as tea to relax and calm the body.	Apply to affected areas (see **CHAMOMILE COMPRESS** recipe page 86). Add 1 teaspoon dried herb or 2 teaspoons fresh herb to hot water and steep for 5 minutes.	None when taken at recommended dosage.
	chaste tree berry *(Vitex agnus-castus)*	Hormone-balancing restorative herb used to treat PMS or menopause.	Take in liquid tincture or capsule form alone or with other skin-clarifying herbs.	In tincture form, add 2 ml (50 drops) twice daily to juice or water. In capsule form, take 400 mg daily or as directed by physician.	Avoid during pregnancy and while nursing.
	dandelion root *(Taraxacum officinalis)*	Liver tonic herb used to detoxify entire system.	Take in liquid tincture or capsule form alone or with other skin-clarifying herbs.	In tincture form, add 2 ml (50 drops) twice daily to juice or water. In capsule form, take 200 mg daily or as directed by physician.	Avoid during pregnancy and while nursing.
	evening primrose *(Oenothera biennis)*	Effective skin-soothing herb due to high gamma-linolenic acid content.	Take in capsule form or use externally in cream or ointment.	Take 500 mg twice daily or as directed by physician to promote healthy skin.	None at recommended dose.

HERB	BENEFITS	APPLICATIONS	INSTRUCTIONS	PRECAUTIONS
green tea *(Camellia sinensus)*	Antioxidant used to fight free radicals.	Drink as tea.	Add 1 teaspoon dried herb to hot water and steep for 5 minutes. Drink 4 or 5 cups daily.	Contains a small amount of caffeine.
milk thistle *(Silybum marianum)*	Cleansing herb for liver and gallbladder.	Take in liquid tincture or capsule form alone or with other skin-clarifying herbs.	In tincture form, take 2 ml (50 drops) 3 times daily; In capsule form, take 250 mg daily or as directed by physician.	None when taken at recommended dosage.
oat seed *(Avena sativa)*	Anti-inflammatory herb calms red, itchy skin conditions.	Use externally to calm irritated skin (See **PLANT MILK** recipe page 78). Use internally in liquid tincture or capsule form as nerve tonic.	In tincture form, add 2 ml (50 drops) twice daily to juice or water. In capsule form, take 200 mg daily or as directed by physician.	None when taken at recommended dosage.
psyllium husk	Aids in sluggish digestion.	Take in capsule form to keep intestines clear.	Take 1000 mg with a minimum of 8 ounces water.	Avoid during pregnancy. Drink plenty of water.
red clover *(Trifolium pretense)*	Blood purifier and skin-soothing herb, especially irritated skin such as eczema or psoriasis.	Take in liquid tincture or capsule form alone or with other skin-clarifying herbs.	In tincture form, take 2 ml (50 drops) 3 times daily; In capsule form, take 200 mg daily or as directed by physician.	None when taken at recommended dosage.
stevia	Sweetener.	Add to teas or liquid tinctures to sweeten.	$1/4$ teaspoon stevia is equivalent to 1 teaspoon sugar.	None when taken at recommended dosage.
valerian *(Valeriana officinalis)*	Sedative herb is useful in promoting sleep.	Take in liquid tincture or capsule form to calm the nerves and promote sleep.	In tincture form, take 2 ml (50 drops) before bedtime. In capsule form, take 200 mg before bedtime.	Causes drowsiness; do not drive or operate machinery when taking.

HERBAL PRESCRIPTIONS

The following recipes provide solutions to everyday skin-care complaints. Use them to supplement your personalized beauty-care regimen.

HEALING CALENDULA SALVE

SKIN PERSONALITY

B   HR   SR   ER   M

MAKES ½ OUNCE

PREP TIME:
30 MINUTES

This all-natural version of Bag Balm, a well-known farmers salve, is perfect for dry, irritated, or chapped skin. CALENDULA is traditionally known as a wound healer and its anti-inflammatory properties make it excellent for eczema, psoriasis, acute dermatitis, or a wound or burn. The BEESWAX base is quickly absorbed into the skin, leaving your skin smooth and soft without the greasy feel that petrochemical bases such as mineral oil and paraffin leave behind.

½ ounce Calendula Infused Oil (see page 67)
½ tablespoon grated beeswax
3 drops German chamomile
    (*Chamomile Matricaria recutita*) essential oil
2 drops lavender (*Lavandula vera*) essential oil

½-ounce glass ointment jar

Place Calendula Infused Oil and beeswax in a heatproof glass measuring cup. Place cup in a shallow pan of simmering water. Heat, stirring constantly, until all of the ingredients are melted together. Add chamomile and lavender essential oils and stir until well mixed. Pour into ointment jar and place in the refrigerator to set. Apply liberally to body as needed.

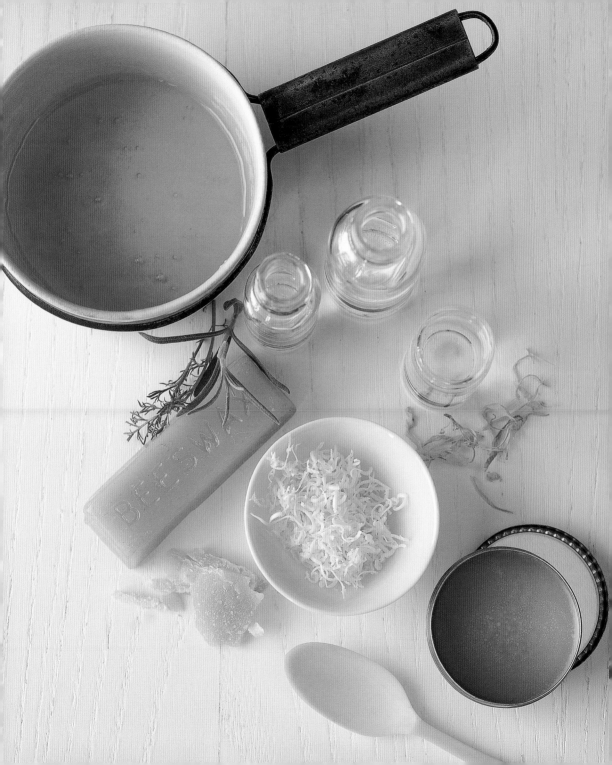

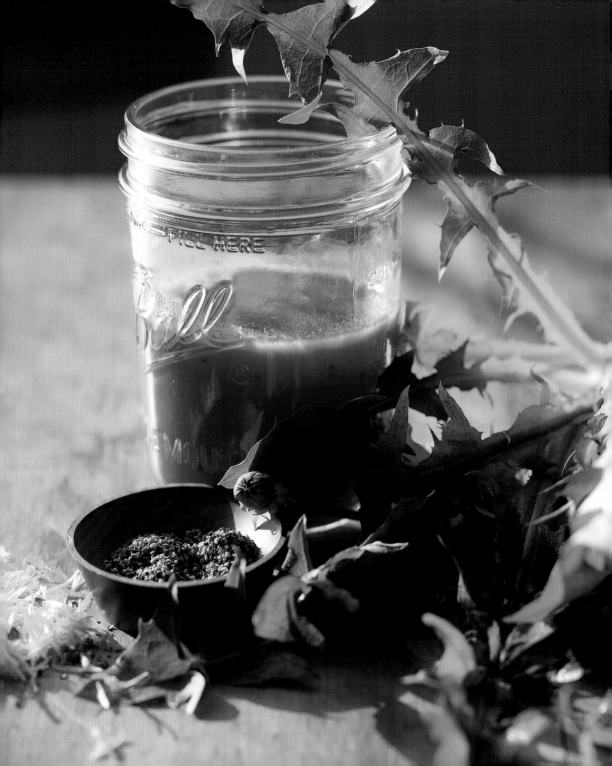

DANDELION DETOX DRINK

Tomato juice, fortified with the antioxidant LYCOPENE, is excellent for a sluggish liver, and the LEMON JUICE helps to alkalinize the blood. This remedy is also a great hangover cure, since the fructose helps to correct your blood sugar and assists your body in metabolizing alcohol faster.

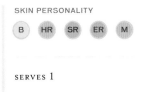
1 cup tomato juice
⅛ teaspoon Worcestershire sauce
⅛ teaspoon horseradish
1 tablespoon lemon juice
freshly ground pepper
30 to 60 drops dandelion tincture

Combine all ingredients in a canning jar, close, and shake well. Drink 2 to 3 times daily.

COMPLEXION TEA

This clarifying tea is excellent for hormone-reactive skin, since red clover is an effective blood-cleansing herb. Red clover grows in clumps in many fields and meadows in North America. This hardy perennial is easy to recognize by its flower, which varies from pink to rose in hue. Alternatively, you can find red clover at your health food store.

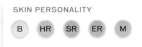
½ cup fresh red clover blossoms
1 teaspoon dried rose hips
1 teaspoon shredded lemon peel
2 teaspoons chopped fresh peppermint leaves
2 cups purified water

Combine the first four ingredients in a French press. Pour in boiling water and let tea steep for 10 minutes. For acute skin breakouts, drink 4 cups a day until symptoms abate.

SOOTHING BURDOCK SOUP

SKIN PERSONALITY

B HR SR ER M

MAKES 6 SERVINGS

PREP TIME:
90 MINUTES

BURDOCK ROOT is indispensable for soothing hot, itchy, or inflamed skin. It is an excellent remedy to use when the skin feels fiery, such as during episodes of eczema, psoriasis, or rashes and is therefore an herbal ally for stress-reactive and environment-reactive skin personalities. Burdock is a blood purifier and so is also a good friend to hormone-reactive skin personalities. It is a nourishing skin tonic, fortified with high levels of iron, magnesium, and vitamins A and C. Burdock root can be found at any health food store or Japanese market. Or, if you are feeling ambitious, go for a weed walk. If you have ever spent time on a farm you may recognize burdock as a tall, spiky plant with purple thistle flowers. Burdock root is best in the fall, on two-year-old plants whose thistle flowers have turned to brown burrs.

1 cup chopped onion
2 cloves garlic, minced
1 cup chopped fresh burdock root
1 cup peeled and sliced carrots
1 pound potatoes (russet or wax)
½ cup fresh dandelion leaves (optional)
6 cups vegetable stock or water
Salt
3 tablespoons dry white wine or sherry
3 tablespoons chopped parsley

Combine vegetables and stock in pot and bring to a boil. Add salt to taste, reduce heat, and cover, simmering for 1 hour. Remove 2 cups of soup, puree in a blender, and return to pot. Stir in sherry and parsley and simmer for 20 more minutes.

PEACEFUL SLEEP TEA

This recipe contains CHAMOMILE, a gentle, relaxing herb that is
also good for upset stomachs. What makes this tea especially effective
at bringing on sleep is VALERIAN, a potent nerve tonic. Drink this tea
1 hour before bedtime.

SKIN PERSONALITY

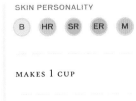

MAKES 1 CUP

PREP TIME:
10 MINUTES

> 1 cup purified water
> ½ teaspoon chamomile flowers
> 30 to 40 drops valerian tincture

Pour boiling water over chamomile flowers in a French press. Steep
for 5 minutes. Strain and add valerian tincture.

ICED FIJI GREEN TEA

Green tea is brimming with cancer-fighting antioxidants that help wipe
out free radicals, which can damage skin on the cellular level. Drink
this beverage throughout the day to help maintain optimal skin fitness.

SKIN PERSONALITY

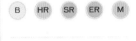

MAKES 1 GALLON

PREP TIME:
15 MINUTES

> 1 gallon purified water
> 1 ounce Fiji green tea or other fine Sencha green tea
> 1 gallon of purified water
> ½ cup unsweetened apple or white grape juice
> Crushed ice

In a saucepan bring water to a rolling boil and remove from heat.
Place green tea inside tea infusion ball and immerse in water for 2
to 3 minutes or according to taste. Remove infusion ball and let tea
cool. Pour juice into a gallon-sized glass container with a lid, add
green tea, close lid, and shake. Refrigerate. Pour tea infusion over
ice into glass.

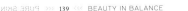

ENERGETIC MEDICINES

Equally important in the herbal skin-care pharmacy are energetic medicines such as homeopathic remedies and flower essences. Homeopathic remedies are especially useful in skin-care problems because their subtle vibrational energies work well with chronic complaints that allopathic medicines fail to treat.

HOMEOPATHY

Homeopathy is the second most widely used system of medicine in the world and is based on three principles:

"LIKE CURES LIKE." For example, if the symptoms of your insomnia are similar to those of ingesting too much caffeine, then coffee might be your homeopathic remedy.

MINIMAL DOSE. The remedy is taken in an extremely dilute form; normally 1 part remedy to around 1,000,000,000,000 parts water. These dosages are delivered on a sugar tablet and are taken under the tongue.

THE SINGLE REMEDY. No matter how many symptoms are experienced, only one remedy is taken, and that remedy will be aimed at all of the symptoms.

Some homeopathic remedies are particularly useful for skin care. *Arnica Montana* aids in the speedy healing of bruises. *Calcarea Sulphurica* soothes irritated skin conditions such as acne, boils, eczema. *Coffee Cruda* counters insomnia from stress or an overactive mind. *Thuja Occidentalis* is used for acne, dandruff, and fungal viruses such as warts. *Utica Urens* is an antidote to hives, sunburns, and rashes. For each ingest 6c or 30c under tongue, as directed by the manufacturer.

FLOWER ESSENCES

The use of flower essences is based on somewhat the same principles as homeopathy but focuses more on imbalances of an emotional nature, so flower essences are useful for stress-related problems. The most popular flower essences are the Bach flower essences, discovered in the 1930s by Dr. Edward Bach. Bach flower essences are composed of thirty-eight homeopathically prepared remedies, which represent a complete system of healing directed at the personality, mood, and emotional outlook of an individual.

The best flower essence cure to take for skin-care related problems is Rescue Remedy, a combination of essences including Cherry Plum, Clematis, Impatiens, Rock Rose, and Star of Bethlehem. Rescue Remedy helps to calm the mind. Visit the Bach Flower Web site at www.bachessences.com to learn about creating the flower essence that would best suit your skin personality.

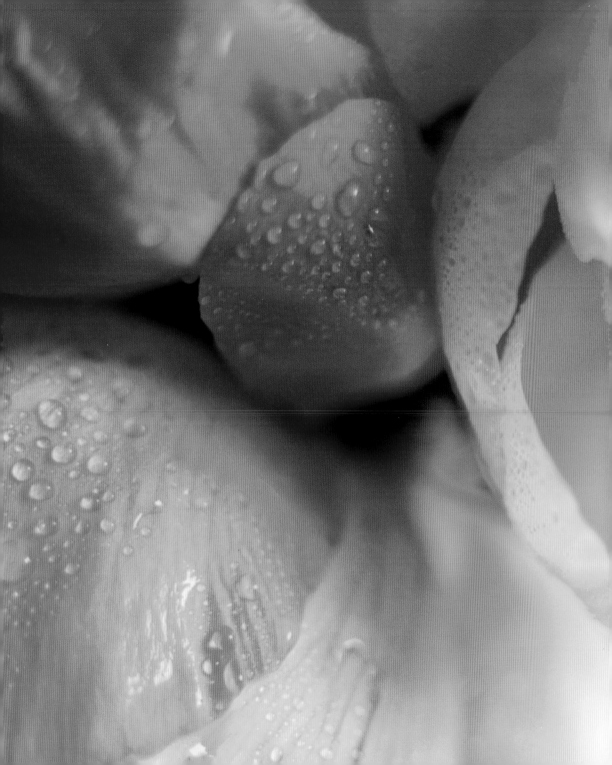

RESOURCES

Botanical Skin-Care Products, Essential Oils, Cosmetic Materials, and Herbal Remedies

Aphrodesia Herb Shoppe
264 Bleecker Street
New York, NY 10014
212.989.6440
Large assortment of base skin-care materials and herbal ingredients.

Avena Botanicals
219 Mill Street
Rockport, ME 04856
207.594.0694
High-quality dried herbs and tinctures, oils, salves. Catalog.

The Fragrant Earth Co., Ltd
Glastonbury, BA69EW
United Kingdom
360.651.9809
(U.S.A. inquiries)
www.fragrant-earth.com
Essential oils and cosmetic raw materials. Catalog.

Naturopathica
74 Montauk Highway
East Hampton, NY 11937
800.669.7618
www.naturopathica.com
Botanical skin-care, herbal remedies, essential oils, herbal and vegetal carrier oils, herbal teas. Catalog.

Original Swiss Aromatics
P.O. Box 6723
San Rafael, CA 94903
415.479.9121
www.originalswissaromatics.com
Comprehensive selection of premium essential oils.

Prima Fleur Botanicals
1525 East Francisco Boulevard, Suite 16
San Rafael, CA 94901
415.455.0957
www.primafleur.com
Essential oils, cosmetic raw materials. Catalog.

Trinity Herbs
P.O. Box 100
Graton, CA 95444
707.824.2040
Herbs, tinctures, teas, beeswax.

Bottles and Jars

O. Berk Company
Union, NJ 07083
908.851.9500
www.oberk.com
Large cosmetic packaging supplier.

SKS Bottle & Packaging
3 Knabner Road
Mechanicville, NY 12118
518.899.7488
www.sks-bottle.com
Supplier of glass and plastic bottles, cosmetic jars, atomizers, etc.

Holistic Lifestyle Products

Cutting Edge Catalog
P.O. Box 4158
Santa Fe, NM 87501
800.497.9516
www.cutcat.com
Holistic lifestyle catalogue.

Gaiam
360 Interlocken Boulevard
Broomfield, CO 80021
877.989.6321
www.gaiam.com
This is a complete resource for a holistic lifestyle. The catalog contains shower filters, air purifiers, and humidifiers as well as yoga and fitness products, nontoxic household cleaners, and more.

Multi-Pure Water Filters
7251 Cathedral Rock Drive
Las Vegas, NV 89128
800.622.9206
www.multipure.com
High-quality water filters.

Organizations and Educational Resources

AlternativeMedicine.com
1650 Tiburon Boulevard
Tiburon, CA 94920
800.515.4325
www.alternativemedicine.com
Huge database of alternative medicine information.

American Academy of
Dermatology
P.O. Box 4014
930 North Meachum Road
Schaumburg, IL 60168
847.330.0050
www.aad.org

Resources for Finding
Qualified Dermatologists,
Skin Care Articles, and
Related Information

American Association of
Naturopathic Physicians
(AANP)
3201 New Mexico Avenue NW,
Suite 350
Washington, D.C. 20016
866.538.2267
www.naturopathic.org
Good resource for finding qualified
naturopathic doctors, natural health
publications, and information.

The American Botanical
Council
6200 Manor Road
Austin, TX 78723
www.herbalgram.com
Complete resource on herbal medicine,
safety guidelines, periodicals, etc.

Bach Flower Essences
www.bachessences.com
Visit this Web site to learn to create
your own customized flower essence
to fit your skin personality.

Glycemic Index Online
www.glycemicindex.com
Web resource for information on high
glycemic foods and how to monitor them.

REFERENCES

Boyle, Wade, and Andre Saine. *Lectures in Naturopathic Hydrotherapy.* East Palestine, Ohio: Buckeye Naturopathic Press, 1988.

Brewer, Sarah. *The Total Detox Plan.* London: Carlton Books Limited, 2000.

Erickson, Kim. *Drop-Dead Gorgeous.* New York: McGraw-Hill Company, 2002.

Hampton, Aubrey. *What Is in Your Cosmetics?* New York: Odonian Press, 1995.

Michalun, Natalia, and M. Varinia Michalun. *Milady's Skin Care & Cosmetic Ingredients Dictionary.* New York: Delmar, 2001.

Null, Gary. *The Complete Guide to Health and Nutrition.* New York: Dell, 1984.

_____. *Get Healthy Now! A Complete Guide to Prevention, Treatment and Healthy Living.* New York: Seven Stories Press, 1999.

Perricone, Nicholas. *The Perricone Prescription.* New York: HarperCollins Publishers, 2002.

Schnaubelt, Kurt. *Advanced Aromatherapy.* Rochester, Vt.: Healing Arts Press, 1998.

_____. *Medical Aromatherapy: Healing with Essential Oils.* Berkeley, CA: Frog Ltd, c/o North Atlantic Books, 1999.

Steinman, David, and Samuel S. Epstein. *The Safe Shopper's Bible: A Consumer's Guide to Nontoxic Household Products, Cosmetics, and Food.* New York: Wiley Publishing Inc., 1995.

Weil, Andrew. *Eight Weeks to Optimum Health: A Proven Program for Taking Full Advantage of Your Body's Natural Healing Power.* New York: Alfred A. Knopf, 1997.

Winter, Ruth. *A Consumer's Dictionary of Cosmetic Ingredients,* New York: Three Rivers Press, 1999.

Worwood, Valerie Ann. *The Complete Book of Essential Oils and Aromatherapy.* London: New World Library, 1991.

_____. *Aromatherapy for the Beauty Therapist.* London: Thompson, 2001.

INDEX